Breathe, Focus, Excel

Exercises, Techniques, and Strategies for Optimal Athletic Performance

Harvey Martin

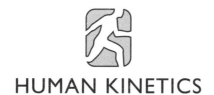

HUMAN KINETICS

Library of Congress Cataloging-in-Publication Data

Names: Martin, Harvey, 1989- author.
Title: Breathe, focus, excel : exercises, techniques, and strategies for
    optimal athletic performance / Harvey Martin.
Description: Champaign, IL : Human Kinetics, [2024] | Includes
    bibliographical references.
Identifiers: LCCN 2022038350 (print) | LCCN 2022038351 (ebook) | ISBN
    9781718210172 (paperback) | ISBN 9781718210189 (epub) | ISBN
    9781718210196 (pdf)
Subjects: LCSH: Respiratory organs--Physiology. | Breathing exercises. |
    Sports--Physiological aspects. | BISAC: HEALTH & FITNESS / Exercise /
    General | HEALTH & FITNESS / Healthy Living & Personal Hygiene
Classification: LCC RC1236.R47 M37 2024 (print) | LCC RC1236.R47 (ebook)
    | DDC 613/.192--dc23/eng/20220929
LC record available at https://lccn.loc.gov/2022038350
LC ebook record available at https://lccn.loc.gov/2022038351

ISBN: 978-1-7182-1017-2 (print)

Senior Acquisitions Editor: Michelle Earle; **Developmental Editor:** Laura Pulliam; **Managing Editor:** Shawn Donnelly; **Copyeditor:** Annette Pierce; **Permissions Manager:** Laurel Mitchell; **Senior Graphic Designer:** Joe Buck; **Cover Designer:** Keri Evans; **Cover Design Specialist:** Susan Rothermel Allen; **Photograph (cover):** PeopleImages / Getty Images; **Photograph (title page):** olegganko/Adobe Stock; **Photographs (interior):** © Human Kinetics, unless otherwise noted; photos on pages 185, 186, and 188 © **Nolan Johnson;** photo on page 182 © Ryan Rourk; **Photo Production Specialist:** Amy M. Rose; **Photo Production Manager:** Jason Allen; **Senior Art Manager:** Kelly Hendren; **Illustrations:** © Human Kinetics, unless otherwise noted; **Printer:** Versa Press

We thank MASH Performance in Eagan, Minnesota, for assistance in providing the location for the photo shoot for this book.

Human Kinetics books are available at special discounts for bulk purchase. Special editions or book excerpts can also be created to specification. For details, contact the Special Sales Manager at Human Kinetics.

Printed in the United States of America

10 9 8 7 6 5 4 3 2 1

The paper in this book is certified under a sustainable forestry program.

Human Kinetics
1607 N. Market Street
Champaign, IL 61820
USA

United States and International
Website: **US.HumanKinetics.com**
Email: info@hkusa.com
Phone: 1-800-747-4457

Canada
Website: **Canada.HumanKinetics.com**
Email: info@hkcanada.com

E8463

To my parents, Jim and Karen, who have been with me since the beginning, always standing behind me as I've pursued my passions and curiosity in life. And to my love, Chelsea—the one who has supported me on every step of the journey and been a true, constant source of inspiration.

–Love, Harvey

Contents

Exercise Finder

Foreword

Historically, mental skills in sports are difficult to study and quantify. Breathing, meditation, and hot/cold modalities are well researched, however, and proven for performance enhancement, stress reduction, a clearer mindset, and a way to build energy or to come down from an adrenaline surge. Breath training has science and research behind it. It's not top secret, but it's underutilized as a technique.

Hunting for a mental skills coach is a challenge. And while Harvey isn't a mental skills coach in the traditional sense, he's an innovative, fresh perspective type of thinker. In order to be a good coach or staff member in the clubhouse, it's really helpful to be a good listener. Before Harv is coaching, teaching, or sharing information, he's listening. He listens to athletes and learns what they need in the way of support to be great.

Harv is an evidence-based dude, and evidence is important when it comes to asking athletes to change their routine. They need to know that there is something behind this change, not just "hey, I think this might work." It's less trial and error and more research-and-development-based suggestions for our players. It's easy to find good content in baseball and in sports. It's more difficult to find the vehicle to deliver it, and Harvey has a unique ability to deliver content.

We are really happy we have him.

—Gabe Kapler, Major League Manager, San Francisco Giants

Preface

It was early December of 2015, and I had been released from professional baseball a few months before with something athletes and coaches call the yips. The yips are a feeling similar to a minor panic attack that you experience while performing. My case of the yips came while throwing a baseball, and because I was a pitcher, this was not a positive experience. I would feel frozen, tight, and heavy when I picked up a ball to play catch. The result would be wild throws, mass confusion, and depression. The yips, however, are not unique to baseball, but can be experienced in other sports and activities: free throw shooting in basketball, putting in golf, singing at an audition. The ability to move and think suddenly becomes frozen.

I, like many athletes whose careers end abruptly, felt lost. Troubled by the lack of finances that come with playing minor league sports, I moved to Minnesota, where I had played college baseball a few years earlier. I wasn't able to afford rent or buy a place of my own; however, I had a mattress that fit perfectly inside a friend's closet. I called this closet home for a little over a year as I slowly picked up the pieces, changed careers, and started the process of creating a new life. At the time, I was confused, upset, and lost because my lifelong dream had come to an end and, for the first time in my life, I didn't have a purpose. On top of all this, on a yearly basis, I experienced strep throat, nasal congestion, a constant dry mouth while sleeping, and frequent nighttime trips to the bathroom to urinate. In the midst of sleepless nights and feelings of hopelessness, I had become a former athlete with a lost identity who was also battling chronic illness.

Little did I know that my life would change in just a matter of months after being released from sport. I met a yogi, began a 16-week process of focused meditation, and took cold showers—a combination rarely advised in modern-day athletic programs. My instructions were simple: Get back to nature, and breathe. My goal was to learn about breathing, control my mind, and improve my health—exactly what the yogi instructed. After 16 weeks of breath work, my final test would be to take everything I had learned and practiced while confronting one of my greatest fears: deep bodies of water in nature coupled with extreme cold temperatures.

As part of this process, I learned that most people breathe vertically into their auxiliary breathing muscles (the neck, shoulders, and upper chest), constricting the vagus nerve. The vagus nerve, which will be discussed in more detail later in the book, plays a crucial role in activating the parasympathetic nervous system, which controls involuntary functions and is involved in rest and digestion. It also affects blood pressure and heart rate. All play a critical role in an athlete's ability to generate healthy adaptations. These poor breathing mechanics can result in a constant state of anxiety, which disrupts the ability to adapt to stress and reduces the ability to reach full potential in recovery and mental focus. Through this process, I found out I was a vertical breather.

Learning to breathe into the middle of the body, rather than into the upper chest and neck, is crucial for the modern athlete. Not only does it improve your power output by creating core stability, but it also allows fluid breathing rhythms for your mind to follow. Your brain constantly spies on the way you breathe and is always relaying information. For example, your breathing adjusts by speeding up when you're anxious or exercising and by slowing down when you're asleep.

Why would this be important for athletes to know? Breathing underlies all aspects of brain function and controls the state of the nervous system. If you find yourself chronically overbreathing, breathing quickly and shallowly, your brain shuts down important aspects of performance, such as controlling motor skills and thinking clearly. As I began to understand this, I learned that my performance anxiety and inability to throw a baseball were caused by my lack of awareness of how I was breathing. When I first began breathwork, I needed to grasp the mechanics of breathing by learning how to engage the diaphragm; soon, I learned to breathe slowly in a neutral position with a tall spine. By creating habits of breathing slowly and fully, you can begin to incorporate specific breathing practices and breath-holding exercises. Over time, you notice the changes occurring in the mind and body.

I practiced these methods during my 16 weeks of focused breath training. As the yogi instructed, I became aware—to feel and learn my body from within. My daily practice of deep breathing and mindful focus would eventually be tested. In mid-December when I took the plunge and sunk into the depths of a frozen lake, I felt present for the first time in my life. Future worries disappeared, and guilt no longer anchored me down. All those months of confusion and uncertainty eventually led to a moment of bliss, a moment that forever changed my life. After that pivotal day, I found myself routinely holding my breath for over three minutes and comfortably carving holes in the ice so I could sit in Minnesota's frozen lakes. I was told this process would change my life. And sure enough, it did. I achieved a goal that had felt unattainable a few short months earlier and brought happiness back into my life after the end of my baseball career. The only change I made was to learn my breathing and get into nature.

From here I made a choice to understand the depths of the breath. How was I able to control my state in cold water? Why did my anxieties go away? Why was I no longer urinating in the middle of the night or waking up to drink water to wet my palate? My strep throat seemed to be gone for good and my allergies minimized, with little to no nasal congestion. I packed my bags and started traveling. I learned from breath masters around the world and earned certifications in the mechanics of breathing and the physiological and psychological connection of breathing. I also studied the effects of heat and cold exposure, known as environmental stress, on the body and how this affects the cells and tissue quality as well as state of mind. I learned movement practices and yoga techniques to comfortably control the breath, improve lung capacity, and strengthen my endurance. After my studies, I began training small groups and then larger groups and eventually professional athletes and teams.

In this book, I want you to harness the power of your breath so you can use it to begin your path toward reaching your full potential—like I did when I plunged into that freezing lake. That cold December winter in Minnesota taught me some of my greatest lessons: Stay calm, focus your breathing, trust yourself, and control what you can control.

If you want to maximize your athletic performance, this book will help you understand that the answer lives within you—it's in your breath. Inside these chapters, you will learn the history and science behind breath work and how it can change your game. You will learn mechanical movements that expand the rib cage, protect the spine, and strengthen the pelvic floor, allowing you to move and recover better. You will improve your aerobic capacity so you can go farther with less effort and gain an edge in the clarity of your thinking and decision-making. Enjoy the journey.

Acknowledgments

I would like to thank the entire organization of Human Kinetics, who took a chance on me and published this book. Thank you to Michelle Earle and Laura Pulliam for their steadfast support and sticking with me throughout the process. I am forever grateful to the San Francisco Giants organization and the leadership of Gabe Kapler and Dave Groeschner, who gave me the opportunity to expand my teachings in sport with the freedom to complete this book. Thank you to all the members of the MindStrong Project, a team of curious individuals who sought to enhance the human experience. Without the connection and commitment from all of you, the principles and lessons within this book would not be possible. I will cherish our friendship and memories forever.

A special thank you to Dana Santas for bringing me this opportunity; without you none of this would be possible. Thank you to all of the teachers, doctors, coaches, and trainers who gave me their time and shared information through interviews and meetings. Every minute of discussion and thought-provoking experience we shared has its imprints within the pages of this book. Thank you to those who gave me their time with dedicated one-on-one coaching and teaching the importance of breath. A special thank you to my early teachers who are all recognized within the book: Dr. Belisa, Brian Mackenzie, Rob Wilson, and Dr. McKeown. I will forever be a student to the field of human performance; thank you for building the classroom.

Part I
Breath Awareness

1

Fundamentals of Breath Awareness

Oxygen is the key to energy production. It's the molecule the body uses to metabolize food to create the energy that fuels all our vital functions. Without energy we are nothing, and our ability to manipulate our breathing to control our mental and physical energy separates us from other life forms, leading to our place at the top of the food chain. However, modern society has pulled us away from our natural state, which has negatively affected how we breathe, which in turn negatively affects our overall well-being. In this book you will learn how to create a single focus on breathing within your athletic training. By learning the tools and being able to implement them, you will see just how powerful breathing is for the advancement of athletic performance.

Breath is the foundation of everything we do. It is the communicator in the mind–body connection and a direct gateway to the nervous system. Breathing is the key to all biological processes in the body. We receive continuous feedback from sensations, perceptions, feelings, and emotions. Functions in the mind and body affect the way we breathe, or the way we breathe affects functions in our mind and body. How we experience reality is a two-way street. Understanding this feedback is the main driver in an athlete's mental and physical state during performance. Breathing can be improved, strengthened, and trained just like any other skill developed on the field or in the weight room. By implementing breath work as a stand-alone practice, athletes have the ability to use breath to affect other components of performance, such as how they move, digest food, recover, sleep, and think. This book teaches how to alter and manipulate respiration to manage energy, understand stress, and adapt to stress.

Throughout the book, you will learn many styles of breathing. In the early chapters, you will learn about chronic mouth breathing and the anatomy, physiology, and psychology of breathing. You will learn how modern lifestyles can disrupt health and how to combat poor breathing and an unhealthy lifestyle by establishing proper breathing mechanics. Mechanics are the motor skills that control the movement of muscles with the intent to perform a specific act. Athletes practice repetitions of the motor skills needed in their sport so they can trust these skills when it matters most. In this book, you will learn how to practice the motor skills necessary for proper respiration.

Breathing is the most basic movement a body performs, and the rest of the body builds on it. It's also a constant—we are always breathing, so it always affects how we move and live. This makes breathing the foundation for all complex movement patterns we make. Strong functional breathing is the base of physical health and longevity.

Because breathing is constant, it is automatic, and we do not have to be conscious of it. This is why it's easy to remain unaware of our breath and let it slip into habitual poor patterns that decrease our well-being over time. However, we can build practices and intention behind our breathing to enhance health and create strong automatic breathing habits without consciously controlling it. This is difficult at first because we lack nerve endings around our diaphragm, which means we don't necessarily feel the diaphragm working or being trained like we do when we work the biceps or hamstrings. This book will help you strengthen the muscles and become aware of how to properly move while you breathe. Be assured that elite athletes are doing this type of breath work. By integrating it into your athletic training, you will raise the ceiling on your potential.

Improving Your Breath

As you start to understand your breath and how you can use it in your athletic performances, you must start with awareness. As an athlete and high-level performer, your main objective is to improve. What you can measure, you can progress, and as humans progress in activities, they go back to them. Think of a person starting a weightlifting program who finds immediate results in that process. As their muscles grow, they find the weight room less intimidating and more attractive, making it easier to continue and to improve.

So how do you create progress in your breathing? Start with the diaphragm. It's the key muscle used in breathing and needs to be worked just like any other muscle, but working this muscle can be frustrating because you can't see or feel that it grew like you can with the biceps after a series of curls. Therefore, you must go deeper into how you perceive progress in breathing.

Breathing, like anything else that athletes do, is a skill. We can improve our breathing, just as we can improve our squat. The beauty of breath practice, however, is that it is more than a mechanical skill. It also contributes to improvements in overall health. In recent years, we have learned that practicing breathing can control our autonomic nervous system, which regulates involuntary processes. Control over this system allows us to regulate other automatic systems in our body, such as heart rate, digestion, and blood circulation. All of these play a tremendous role in our health and natural ability to build immunity. By mastering the breath, we can take ownership of our health, which is a human superpower.

Beyond improving the mechanics of physical performance, breathing gives us direct access to our brain. Three main systems in the brain are directly affected by the breath: the brainstem, which is the most ancient part of the brain; the limbic system, which controls the emotional center of the brain; and the prefrontal cortex, which is responsible for reasoning, problem-solving, comprehension, impulse control, creativity, and perseverance—the things that make us human and separate us from other animals (see figure 1.1).

Regulation of breathing is an instinctual function that takes place in the brainstem and is mainly unconscious. Its main role is to keep the body at homeostasis, which is keeping the physiological systems in balance. Although the involuntary mechanism of breath control is not entirely understood, we know it involves neural signals in respiratory centers that are located in the medulla and pons, which sit just above the spinal cord. These centers control the movement and timing of the breath as well as the rhythm. Overall, this area of the brain fine-tunes the ventilation rate. The respiratory center in the brainstem is affected by high levels of carbon dioxide and low pH, which will be discussed further in chapter 3. These levels are why this area of the brain focuses on homeostasis. If the body feels out of sync, the areas in the brainstem will work to correct that.

The limbic system generates emotional ripple effects that are affected by the way we breathe. Shallow, rapid, inefficient breathing can put us in a weakened, reactionary state where we can't control our emotions. Deep, slow breathing can create a controlled, responsive state where we have a grip on our emotions.

Finally, the prefrontal cortex, which is where decision-making and reasoning take place, allows for voluntary and intentional control of breathing. Voluntary control moves breathing from an unconscious state to a conscious state. This is where breathing becomes the ultimate separator in human evolution: We have the unique ability to control our lives by how we breathe.

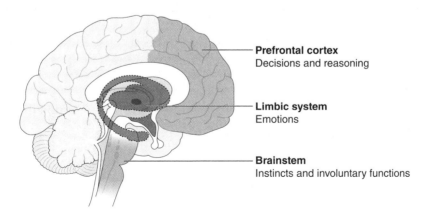

Prefrontal cortex
Decisions and reasoning

Limbic system
Emotions

Brainstem
Instincts and involuntary functions

FIGURE 1.1   The three main systems of the brain.

When we focus on our breath, we start to control our ability to think better, and thinking better gives us, as athletes, a competitive advantage. In later chapters we will focus heavily on breath control and ways to alter the mind.

Recognizing Your Breath

If you want to improve your breathing, where do you start? The first step is to recognize your breath. Recognizing your breath has two parts: (1) understanding the objective and (2) learning how to be aware of your breathing. You must first identify *why* you are focusing on your breath so you can better serve yourself and your practice. Then you must learn *how* to focus on the breath. As an athlete, you have many intentions behind your breath practice and will come to the breath for many reasons. No matter where you are mentally or physically, you must first build the platform for what you're specifically training when you start your breathing practices. Are you focusing on the mechanics, the physiology, or the psychology of breathing? Knowing the objective will bring awareness to the moment and create purpose behind the practice.

Once you have determined your objective, start your breath practice by becoming aware of your breathing. For example, start by sitting or lying comfortably and placing your attention on the flow of your breath. Focus on the inhalation and exhalation. Notice natural pauses that may take place after an inhalation or exhalation. Do you notice a hesitation with your breathing? Or maybe it's more difficult to exhale than to inhale. The objective is to become aware of the flow of the breath.

Once you've set aside time to follow your breathing in a controlled and comfortable environment, take this new awareness into your everyday life. When you're working, driving in traffic, eating, or spending time in conversation, check back in with your breath. How is the flow related to the situation you're experiencing? In this phase of mindful breathing there is no need for specific answers or any answers at all. You are not trying to improve or question the breath. You're just noticing it.

As you practice bringing awareness to your breath, use these questions to strengthen your understanding of your breath:

Nose or Mouth Breathing

Do I breathe through my nose when I'm not training or competing?

Do I experience nasal congestion often?

Sleep

Do I wake up with a dry mouth?

Do I have to get up during the night to drink water or use the bathroom?

Do I snore at night?

Do I have chronic fatigue throughout the day?

Mind

Do I have trouble staying focused on a specific task for an extended period of time?

Do I find myself anxious throughout the day?

Do I have trouble retaining information?

Body

Do I have gut issues?

Do I have trouble controlling my heart rate?

Do I have high blood pressure?

Sound

Can I hear myself breathing while I'm talking?

Can I hear myself breathing while I'm relaxing?

Spend a week answering these questions in a journal at the beginning or end of each day. If you answered *yes* on any day to one of the questions, chances are you were breathing poorly. This book will help you train in those areas. Breathing at rest is meant to be quiet and slow and to flow fluidly solely through the nose. When nasal breathing is disrupted, health within the mind and body will deteriorate and cause unwanted stress. Becoming aware of how you breathe throughout the day is the first step in being able to individualize breathing practice.

It is important to remember that you are breathing during all activities. You are breathing while you rest and during sleep. You are breathing when you are eating or talking. You are also breathing during stressful activities such as arguing, watching a horror movie, or driving at rush hour.

We live in an era of overstimulation, and unwanted stress is a result. Stress affects our breathing, which can trigger the sympathetic nervous system to fire up the fight-or-flight response. Although too much time in an aroused state is detrimental to health, the body and mind need stress to survive, and future chapters will touch on its importance. Elite athletes understand that rapid mouth breathing belongs solely to intense training and competition because that's when they want the mind and body to execute and evolve under stress. Outside of these stressful activities, the mind and body need to adapt and regenerate through slow nasal breathing.

By understanding the activities that call for mouth breathing, athletes are able to maintain health and regenerate outside of training or competition and decrease their levels of stress. The result of stress management is healthy athletes who are able to sustain their careers. Dr. Ross Andel, director of the School of Aging Studies at the University of South Florida, was interviewed in a *Sports Illustrated* article about the 2021 Sportsperson of the Year, Tom

Brady. The article discusses Brady's longevity as an NFL quarterback and the health practices that keep him aging gracefully. "It's the stimulation, the change of environment that challenges the brain and redistributes our bodily resources," says Andel. "He's unbelievably adaptable" (Wertheim 2021).

The ability to adapt to stress will be the edge-chasing formula for elite athletes of the future. According to Robert Sapolsky, the author of *Behave: The Biology of Humans at Our Best and Worst*, we are only about 70 years into understanding that sustained stress can impair our health (2017). And we're becoming aware that modern stressors and overstimulation are the main drivers affecting health today. Humans have always faced stresses such as illness, hunger, working conditions, and the pollution of the industrial age, but athletes are becoming injured and burned out as these factors rise, and the result is a shortened athletic career. Researchers at Sweden's Karolinska Institute studied 680 athletes representing 16 sports. Injuries were a significant problem for elite adolescent athletes (Karolinska Institute 2017). During an average week, one to three athletes were injured. Over a year, almost all of them had been injured at least once, and about 75 percent reported that their injury during the year had been serious.

Through this book, you will learn how to use your breathing to maximize adaptation and decrease injury. You will learn to breathe more effectively during movements to control your physiological and mental processes. You will also learn natural recovery methods to help you become adaptable. Learn and use as many breathing techniques as possible, but keep in mind that it's all about making yourself a more adaptable athlete who can handle stimulation and stress in the modern era.

Understanding the Impact of Mouth Breathing

A major reason modern athletes adapt to stress poorly is because they chronically mouth breathe. As a society, we have become poor breathers, which makes the ancient practice of focused breathing more relevant now than ever before. The rest of this chapter will explain how this has happened. We will learn the difference between mouth and nose breathing, modern life's impact on breathing, how our facial structure affects breathing, and how our breathing relates to sleep.

Mouth Breathing Versus Nose Breathing

Breathing through the mouth and chronically overbreathing, taking shallow or rapid deep breaths, or hyperventilating, send the body into a state of fight or flight that minimizes the healthy exchange of oxygen and carbon dioxide in the body. Alternatively, breathing through the nose instantly lowers the breathing rate, which keeps the body in homeostasis and promotes a more regenerative state. It also directs a better diaphragmatic range, which massages organs and maximizes the exchange of oxygen and carbon dioxide—the main function of breathing (Mayo Clinic n.d.).

The nose is primarily used for breathing, while the mouth is meant for talking and eating. We can breathe through both, but the benefits of nose breathing far outweigh the benefits of breathing through the mouth. The nose brings air deep into the lungs, providing constant positive communication with the brain and supplying a longer-lasting energy. The benefits of nasal breathing include the following (Allen 2015):

- Facilitates correct action of the diaphragm
- Ensures correct position of the tongue (against upper palate) and that lips are closed
- Produces nitric oxide, which opens the blood vessels to help deliver oxygen to muscles
- Prevents pathogens in the air from getting into the bloodstream
- Humidifies the air and warms the flow of oxygen into the lungs
- Increases oxygenation into the muscle tissue by 20 percent
- Reaches lower into the lungs, which provides more oxygen

One important benefit of nose breathing is keeping pathogens from entering the body. When breathing through the nose, the air is slowed and cleaned by the hairs inside the nose and the pathway the air travels through (chapter 2 will cover this function in more depth). The mouth, however, does not provide these defenses. When we breathe through the mouth, there is no protection for the lungs, and we can be at risk from the quality of the air we breathe in. The air we take into our lungs reaches the rest of our body and controls the functions of the cells, and with high-functioning cells, we experience life with more energy.

Breathing through the mouth not only disrupts breathing's filtration system, but it also signals alarm and the need for retreat. Chapter 2 will detail the effect of mouth breathing and the stress response, but for now, to feel its effects, place your hand on your chest and take deep breaths through the mouth. You should feel the upper chest moving, a lack of movement in the diaphragm, and a sense of unease as you continue to breathe deeply through the mouth. The nervous system experiences this as sympathetic activity in the body, and when the nervous system is unable to relax, you enter a chronic sympathetic state that results in a weaker immune system, poor mental state, less energy in competition, injury, and decreased motor skills.

Learning that the body interprets breath through the nose and through the mouth differently might come as a surprise because it's easy to think that breathing is simply breathing. Yet how people feel and how they think stems from the pattern of their breathing. Becoming aware of their breath and recognizing what they're feeling should be a high priority for all athletes.

Mouth Breathing and the Modern Lifestyle

Breathing patterns and mechanical structures of the body change based on the environment we're exposed to. Take the function of the jaw. Modern foods are relatively soft, and some people consume part of their diet through liquids. When our jaws don't have to move as much to chew food, they weaken. This is comparable to losing leg strength if we were to stop walking. When our heads are able to sink into pillows and our spines are compromised during sleep, our breath becomes shallow. This also contributes to mouth breathing at night, which will be discussed in detail later. A key to positive breathing is an open airway and a freely moving rib cage. The ribs need to be able to expand and to stretch both the external and internal muscles located alongside each rib. This provides proper spine alignment and positioning of the body. Then the jaw and palate can support the airways and properly place the tongue.

As a society, we have only recently—within the last few centuries—become mouth breathers, and during that time we've seen a massive change in the human jaw. The speed in which this has taken place has led researchers to believe this change has been too fast to be evolutionary. Research and clinical trials suggest that modern humans are living with poor posture and the way we hold our jaws when not voluntarily moving them (such as when speaking, eating, and especially when sleeping) is one of the main causes of our poor posture (Kahn et al. 2020). The jaw has become narrow, creating crooked teeth and smaller airways. The tongue, which should rest at the roof of the mouth, has slipped into the back of the throat, narrowing airways further and constricting and disrupting airflow. This stems from the way the modern world shapes how we live and changes the way we breathe.

In general, living just isn't as difficult as it used to be. We control the climate of our environment, and most of us have the ability to live in relative comfort most of the time. Our beds and pillows are softer, and chairs and couches support our spines. We live a primarily sedentary life indoors, a lifestyle that our ancestors never experienced. These modern comforts have their benefits; however, they impose a cost to our health. Modern society's health as a whole is experiencing higher rates of anxiety, depression, back pain, and obesity.

When your breathing doesn't feel satisfying or feels restricted, it is telling you that something is off, and it's time to study your environment. Have you recently been startled? Are you surrounded by negativity? Have you been indoors all day? Maybe you have been sitting or lying down for too long? All of these scenarios restrict your breathing. More often than not, your breath will be the first signal that you need to get out, move around, or change your environment.

This is difficult to pick up on if you have not built an awareness of your breathing. In a changing environment, breathing is the only constant. The more you can design an environment that promotes optimal breathing outside of conscious control, the more improvement and adaptation will take place. This means finding time to stand instead of sit, and going on walks and moving rather than sinking into a couch. Also, pay attention to chewing while eating food and take your time during a meal. The jaw muscles gain strength through eating tougher, longer meals. This helps create unconscious nasal breathing and active mindfulness.

By paying attention to your environment, you can avoid long-term health issues stemming from consistent poor breathing. Paul Ehrlich and Daniel Blumstein, authors of "The Great Mismatch," an article on cultural evolution in *BioScience*, stated, "Industrialized humanity has developed an unprecedented lifestyle. Among many other things, that lifestyle has dramatically changed the environments in which humans develop and has led to serious health problems." In their article, they discussed a Stanford University research study that focused on changes in jaw structure since the onset of industrialization and found it was not our genetics leading to a weaker jaw, but our lifestyle. "Assuming that genetics are chiefly responsible for the sudden modern rise of these dental maladies does not make sense," said Ehrlich, a professor of population studies at Stanford. "There's not been enough time for evolution over the span of only several generations to have made our jaws shrink" (Ehrlich and Blumstein 2018). These researchers found that the modern lifestyle and its comforts are disrupting our natural biological processes that keep us healthy.

The Effects of Mouth Breathing

As discussed, our lifestyles have affected our jaw and bone structure, creating a weaker facial structure. The jaw has become narrower, and the face has become longer. This change caused humans to shift from consistent nasal breathers to chronic mouth breathers. You can see it in the faces of people who have weak jaw lines, receding lower jaws, and crooked teeth. Richard Klein, a professor at Stanford University and a paleontologist, is an expert on the human fossil record. In conversation with Paul Ehrlich, who cowrote *Jaws: The Hidden Epidemic* with Sandra Kahn, Klein said, "I've never seen a hunter-gatherer skull with crooked teeth." According to Ehrlich's research, studies of skulls from just a few hundred years ago compared to those of today show that human jaws are shrinking. A few hundred years is not enough time for this to have been caused by genetics. You can't get crowded jaws within a few generations. So it's primarily a response to environmental changes accompanying a sedentary life and industrialization (Kubota 2018).

From early discoveries, we can piece together how distancing ourselves from nature and changing our lifestyle took place. In the 1800s, George Catlin, an adventurer, lawyer, painter, and author, wrote *Shut Your Mouth and Save Your Life*, a book that proposed ideas that at the time seemed far-fetched but have been proven true today. Catlin was searching for answers on why Native Americans had such strong facial features, lived longer, and experienced less illness than white settlers. Catlin's passion for discovery can be traced to his personal life. He spent the majority of his childhood and early adulthood battling illness, and his wife and one of his children died of pneumonia. In his search for why, he noticed that Native Americans slept with their mouths closed. Mothers breastfed their children and made sure the children's lips were sealed together. In early stages, the mothers did this for their children manually until the face muscles grew stronger. Catlin found that Native Americans were training their children to become lifelong nasal breathers.

Catlin visited the gravesites of indigenous tribes and found few children's graves. He compared this to cultures around the world where disease and health issues caused many more deaths in children. From 1830 to 1860, Catlin visited and interviewed more than 150 tribe leaders from North, Central, and South America. He found that the majority of childhood deaths were caused by accidents or natural disasters. The children in the tribes that were not influenced by a European American lifestyle experienced extremely low mortality rates outside of accidents. On the other hand, Catlin found that in Europe during the 1850s, approximately one in four children died at birth, and only one in four survived beyond the age of 25. Poor health was a concern to the people of Europe, but not to Native American tribes.

This convinced him that the cause of diseases in the United States and Europe was not genetics or flaws in physical makeup. These people were dying and experiencing poor mental and physical health because of their lifestyle and habits. Catlin stated, "I am compelled to believe, and feel authorized to assert, that a great proportion of the diseases prematurely fatal to human life, as well as mental and physical deformities, and destruction of the teeth, are caused by the abuse of the lungs, in the Mal-respiration of sleep: and also, that the pernicious habit, though contracted in infancy or childhood, or manhood, may generally be corrected by a steady and determined perseverance, based upon a conviction of its baneful and fatal results." Modern sleep research corroborates this assertion; breathing with the mouth open while sleeping can lead to snoring, and this poor recovery state and low sleep quality eventually cause a decline in overall health.

Breathing is the difference, and Catlin wrote the story that finished in 1870, "Who, like myself, has suffered from boyhood to middle age, everything but death from this enervating and unnatural habit, and then, by a determined and uncompromising effort, has thrown it off, and gained, as it were, a new lease on life and the enjoyment of rest—which have lasted him to an advanced age through exposures and privations, without admitting the mischief of its consequences?" Catlin discovered a few hundred years ago the path we have been headed down, and his contribution to modern health has proven to be significant today.

Both the researchers from Stanford and Catlin's discoveries show that our bodies adapt to the lifestyle we supply it. In the 1960s, a dentist named Egil P. Harvold conducted an experiment with young monkeys by blocking their noses with silicone plugs. The experiment was controversial at the time, and the results were startling. The monkeys developed misalignment of their bite and an elongated lower face that the control monkeys did not (Harvold et al. 1981). This started the conversation on the effects of mouth breathing. The strong evidence from the monkey experiment showed that the body will

The Wandering Nerve

The cranial cavity is dominated by the vagus nerve, which is known as the wandering nerve and plays a major role in our ability to adapt. It runs from the brainstem through the heart and lungs and into the digestive tract and is responsible for regulating the parasympathetic nervous system. The parasympathetic nervous system controls rest and digestion, the sources of regeneration. Consequently, the vagus nerve plays an important role in health. Breathing through the nose tickles this nerve and communicates to the rest of the body the state you're in. You can indirectly stimulate the vagus nerve by taking deep, deliberate breaths through the nose. Deep breathing activates specific neurons that detect functions such as blood pressure. These signals tell the vagus nerve that blood pressure is becoming too high. The vagus nerve responds by lowering the heart rate as you breathe slower and through the nose. Not only does this mitigate the stress response, but it also keeps the body in balance. This is another illustration of the important and deep connection the breath has with the body.

Try this: Place one hand on your belly and the other on your chest. Then do the following:

1. Take five deep breaths through your nose. Make sure you can hear your breathing on both the inhalation and exhalation. The sound will help keep you focused on and mindful of the breath and where in the body the movement occurs.

2. Take five deep breaths through your mouth. Make sure you can hear your breathing on both the inhalation and exhalation. The sound will help keep you focused on and mindful of the breath and where in the body the movement occurs.

You should notice which parts of your body move first and the difference between the first movement in mouth breathing and in nasal breathing. The belly tends to move first and rise with deep nasal breathing. The chest moves first when mouth breathing. This is because mouth breathing uses the upper lungs and nasal breathing uses the lower lungs (closer to the belly). The lower lobes contain the majority of alveoli, the tiny air sacs responsible for the gas exchange of oxygen with carbon dioxide. When you breathe into your upper chest, you access fewer alveoli and pull less oxygen into the body.

adapt to the way we breathe. Children who breathe through their mouth experience the same changes to their facial structure as the monkeys did. Instead of growing forward, the jaw grows backward and downward. This is commonly seen in children who are chronic mouth breathers.

Additional results include the following (Kahn and Ehrlich 2018):

- Weak cheekbones
- Recessed chin
- Negatively tilted eyes
- Convex facial profile
- Flattened midface
- Excess vertical face growth

Daily Habits to Promote Jaw Strength and Nose Breathing

- *Chew gum for 30 minutes a day.* Keep the lips closed and breathe through the nose only. Make sure to chew the gum on both sides of the mouth and keep the teeth together as you swallow.
- *Hold a popsicle stick on one side of the mouth while gently closing down on it.* After 10 minutes, put the popsicle stick on the other side of the mouth as you close down again. Keep your lips closed and breathe through your nose only.
- *Use a jaw exerciser.* Maintain a strong chew habit that strengthens the jaw through practice.
- *Make a fish face.* Pucker your lips and suck in your cheeks for 10 seconds. Relax and repeat 10 to 15 times. Do this three times a day.
- *Massage your face.* Massage along the bones of the entire jaw with just your thumb or with the middle and index fingers together.
- *Practice chin-ups.* Look up toward the ceiling and act as if you're blowing a kiss. You should feel the stretch in the jaw while you hold this position for 30 seconds. Pause and reset. Repeat this 10 times.
- *Stretch your face and move the face muscles.* It may look funny, but open your mouth as wide as you can and move the jaw and facial features around as much as possible until the muscles are fatigued. Repeat 10 times each morning.
- *Repeat A-E-I-O-U.* Saying these letters repeatedly moves the facial features and works the jaw. Say them fast and slow, feeling the changes in the face. Another way to do this is to say one letter and hold that sound for five seconds before saying the next letter.

These structural results have several causes. The face is made up of 42 muscles, and 12 cranial nerves are located in the cranial cavity. These muscles need to be worked and strengthened so they can serve specific functions. Over time, a face with an opened mouth will display narrowed dental arches, referring to the curved shape of the top and bottom set of teeth. A narrowed arch elongates the face because the muscles needed to hold a strong face together are not used. For example, the tongue is meant to rest on the roof of the mouth and should be positioned right behind the top teeth. With the mouth open, the tongue drops down into the bottom of the mouth and closes the airways. The upper dental arch narrows and the midface does not get pushed forward due to the lack of lateral pressure. The lack of muscle use contributes to the poor structure, and the poor structure contributes to further lack of muscle use, resulting in even more shifting.

Can chronic mouth breathing be reversed? The simple answer is yes; however, it is difficult to reverse jaw and bone structure as one gets older. This means that proper breathing habits should be adopted at an early age because children's bones are malleable during growth (see figure 1.2). Ideally, these habits start in infancy. It is suggested that children be breastfed for at least a year because this natural technique allows the child to maintain positive tongue posture and use the muscles in the face to strengthen the jaw. Then, as a developing child continues to grow, it is suggested to lightly pinch the lips together after nursing to encourage nose breathing (Kahn and Ehrlich 2018).

Although you may not be able to change your jaw structure because of the strength of the bones, you have options. The sidebar Daily Habits to Promote Jaw Strength and Nose Breathing offers activities to strengthen the jaw and promote better breathing. You can also use simple tricks to keep

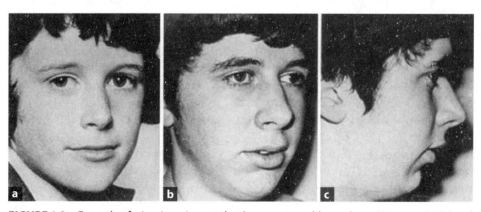

FIGURE 1.2   Example of a jaw impairment that has gone unaddressed over time: age 10 (*a*) and age 17 (*b-c*).

your lips sealed—for example, taping your mouth at night while you sleep or during the day while completing tasks (see the sidebar on the next page). Being aware of keeping the tongue at the roof of the mouth behind the top teeth is important as well. This allows the airways to stay open and promote nasal breathing naturally. Throughout the day pay attention to your lips and keep them gently sealed without the teeth touching.

Mouth Breathing and Sleep

Sleep is becoming a hot topic in modern society. As more than a third of American adults experience poor sleep both in quality and quantity, this is now considered a public health epidemic. Health care practitioners recommend that the average adult needs at least seven hours of sleep each night. Long-term effects of poor sleep are obesity, inactivity, memory loss, and heart disease. And sleep is a top priority in human performance, so it is crucial for improvement and recovery that an athlete sleep well.

Although many factors can cause poor sleep quality and quantity, chronic mouth breathing is one of the biggest reasons. Mouth breathing at rest means we're hyperventilating, which leads to a deficiency in oxygen throughout the body. This causes us to sleep less deeply and keeps the body in a fight-or-flight state.

In a conversation with general dentist Dr. Matt Loomis, Dr. Loomis discussed the dental profession's focus on the airway and its impact on oral and systemic health. Dr. Loomis has seen an increase in patients with cracked teeth, teeth grinding, jaw joint issues, and gum disease. The common denominator for many of these patients isn't obesity, old age, or a poor diet, but rather narrow dental arches, a constricted airway, and the inability to breathe properly through the nose. Dr. Loomis said, "A young 20-year-old track athlete may feel and seem to be in incredible shape; however, if they're snoring at night, this is not normal and they most likely have one or more airway-related issues contributing to this." Dr. Loomis went on to explain that mouth breathing in early age not only weakens the structure of the jaw and disrupts the growth of the teeth, but it also leads to health issues such as hypertension, increased stress, and chronic inflammation throughout the body. Athletes who snore or chronically mouth breathe are not getting the sleep their bodies need to recover and should be evaluated by their dentist or doctor.

When discussing chronic mouth breathing, it is important to mention how modern life and habits affect sleep. The cultural norm of having lightbulbs on during the evening, our lack of sunlight throughout the day, prolonged exposure to computer screens, and highly stressful schedules that keep our systems in a state of chronic stress have become the modern lifestyle. There are many solutions to these problems, and one is to slow the mind and body at

My Mouth-Taping Discovery

It was the fall of 2017, and I was headed to the doctor for a checkup. Assuming I had strep throat, the doctor prescribed antibiotics, and away I went. A few months later my throat collapsed, and I couldn't breathe. I started to have a panic attack as I called a friend to take me to the hospital. A CT scan showed that I had a cyst growing in my throat and needed immediate surgery to cut through the tissue and release the pressure on my arteries.

Eventually my health returned, and I started to regain my strength. However, the last and final issue I was having trouble conquering was sleep. Each night I woke up every few hours with a dry mouth, as cracked as a sidewalk on a hot summer day. I had slept with water next to my bed my entire life, casually waking up to wet my palate when needed. But this time was different. I had never experienced a dryness to the point that my tongue felt heavy to move and it was painful to hydrate.

I decided one night I had to find a way to keep my mouth shut. So I went to the closet and found a piece of tape. That first night I woke up with the tape on my chest, but I noticed something: My tongue wasn't as dry as it had been. I taped up again and slept for a few more hours. Same result, tape on the chest and again less dry. A month into this routine and I started waking up with the tape covering my lips after making it through a full night's sleep. I was breathing through my nose the entire night.

I noticed a few things that changed my life forever. First, I noticed that my mouth had saliva in it when I woke up. My mouth wasn't dry at all, and I eventually stopped putting water at my bedside. Second, I noticed I no longer got up in the middle of the night to use the bathroom. I was neatly tucked into my sheets, just as when I had gotten into bed. My energy skyrocketed, my memory was enhanced, and I felt for the first time that I was truly living. Nasal breathing while I slept had changed the trajectory of my life.

If you're interested in mouth taping or keeping the mouth closed during sleep, be sure to first speak with your doctor to make sure it is safe for you. Here are a few options:

- Mouth tape (Apply petroleum jelly to the lips, and use tape that is strong enough to stay on throughout the course of a night. An Internet search for mouth tape offers numerous options.)
- Nasal strips or nasal dilators
- Antisnore chin strap
- Antisnoring mouthpiece

Be aware that in early use, tape, strips, and mouthpieces may feel uncomfortable or cause anxiety as your body adapts to feeling different during sleep. The mind and body will eventually adapt to this new way of sleeping, you will breathe more slowly during sleep, and the nasal pathways will strengthen through consistent, continuous nasal breathing.

the end of the day with consistent, slow nasal breathing and minimal talking. Slow breathing produces melatonin, a sleep-inducing hormone that improves the recovery and regenerative systems of the body. Less talking keeps the body's oxygen and carbon dioxide exchange in balance. Moreover, focusing attention on these slow breaths reduces anxiety and activates parasympathetic relaxation as the body responds to the slow breathing.

To do this, 10 to 20 minutes before bed, remove yourself from all stimulation (e.g., phone, computer, TV, bright light) and find a comfortable position, either sitting or lying down. Focus the first few moments on the pace of your breath through the nose. After the body feels in rhythm, begin to pause after each inhalation and exhalation. Increase the length of each inhalation and exhalation as you slow the rate of respiration. Specific protocols vary for everyone, but the goal is to slow the breath to promote a sense of relaxation and calmness.

This chapter focused heavily on the negative impact that chronic mouth breathing has on health. Discoveries made hundreds of years ago and more recent findings have given us the insights we need to change our lifestyle. Modern living is easier and much more comfortable than what our ancestors experienced. However, as we expand the comforts of daily life, we must remember that we are humans, walking the planet as an organism that thrives on stress and adaptation. Our biological processes need to experience and adapt to healthy stress, both mental and physical. We are a species meant to breathe through our nose, move all day, and sleep all night. We are meant to follow the natural formula of stress and adaptation.

As you move through this book, maintain a constant awareness of your breath. Take your time with this process and build a relationship with your breathing. You will notice an improvement in the way you move and the strength and endurance you have. More importantly, you will learn how to control arousal, leaving you with a clearer mind and the ability to perform when it matters most. But the first step is to notice your breathing. Keep it simple.

2

The Anatomy and Physiology of Breathing

We learned in chapter 1 that it can be difficult to build awareness of our breathing because it happens automatically. As you take part in breath work or use breathing to control your mind, it helps to have a basic understanding of the anatomy and the physiological processes associated with breathing. This anatomy and physiology of the breath will help you improve more quickly and sustain long-term positive breathing habits so you can compete and perform at the highest level.

The Autonomic Nervous System

The autonomic nervous system plays quite possibly the most important and valuable physiological role in the breathing process, but it's only one part of the larger nervous system (see figure 2.1). The nervous system is divided into the central nervous system (CNS) and the peripheral nervous system (PNS). The central nervous system consists of the brain and spinal cord. The peripheral nervous system includes the cranial nerves and spinal nerves, along with their roots and branches, which are located outside the brain and spinal cord and are responsible for relaying information back to the spinal cord and brain. The PNS is made up of two main functioning systems: the autonomic nervous system (ANS) and the somatic nervous system (SNS). The ANS is responsible for involuntary functions in the body. The SNS is responsible for voluntary actions; it controls muscle movement and uses systems such as the eyes, ears, and skin to send messages to the brain and spinal cord in the central nervous system. All these systems work together to help the mind and body better understand what is going on around us.

The primary purpose of the autonomic nervous system is to regulate the body's internal processes to maintain homeostasis, or physiological equilibrium. This is especially important to athletes. Breathing is the one aspect of the autonomic nervous system that we can consciously control; therefore, it becomes a tool to control the state we desire. But even without our conscious control, our breathing rhythm can naturally change to keep us balanced and

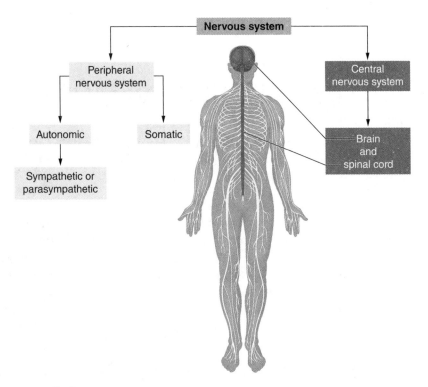

FIGURE 2.1   The human nervous system.

in a state of homeostasis. Think of the last time you felt exhausted during competition or an intense training session. As you felt the stress build up in your body and mind, you most likely recognized how erratic and out of control your breathing felt. Far too often athletes recognize mismanaged breathing too late, which leads to poor performance. To become aware of the breath, athletes need to learn the language of the body and how to manage their energy in order to avoid the risk of breaking down or wanting to quit.

Next time you feel overwhelmed or feel exhaustion starting to set in, pay attention to how fast or hard you're breathing. If it is too difficult to slow your breathing and you're experiencing a high volume of mouth breathing, the nervous system is responding to an overloaded state by relying on the body's reserve systems to try to keep up. The body's reserve fuel tank and how it is affected by erratic breathing will be discussed in chapter 3. In general, you can control erratic breathing by extending the exhalation to double the length of the inhalation. This slows the rate of respiration and signals the nervous system to calm down. Even when breathing through the mouth, this double-length exhalation can return the breathing pattern to normal quickly. This illustrates the ability to consciously control this aspect of homeostasis.

Understanding the Impact of the ANS on Stress and Adaptation

The autonomic nervous system is controlled through two main divisions: the sympathetic and parasympathetic nervous systems. The sympathetic nervous system is said to create a fight-or-flight state; however, a freeze state exists in this system as well. An athlete wants to perform in a "fight" state fueled by an optimal amount of adrenaline. However, the sympathetic nervous system can also create a "flight" or "freeze" state in which the athlete feels fatigued or jittery and makes reactive decisions that impair performance. The parasympathetic nervous system is said to create a rest-and-digest state that is calm and relaxed. The ANS constantly receives information from the external environment and sends feedback to the mind and body based on this information that stimulates the body's processes.

Two simple concepts—stress and adaptation—hold the key to improving athletic performance. Therefore, it is important for athletes to understand how the sympathetic and parasympathetic divisions of the ANS work so they can recognize needed and unneeded stress and then master adaptation. Athletes are between these two states most of the time because they rarely are running for their lives (stress), and they are not spending the day sleeping or digesting food (adapt). Rather, athletes move between the two states numerous times throughout the day, and their breathing responds, depending on which state they are experiencing.

The goal for athletes is to choose the appropriate amount of stress for the appropriate duration in order to maximize adaptation. If there is not enough stress, the athlete can't evolve. Too much stress causes them to break down. The goal is to learn how and when to introduce stress, which requires mastering awareness of the sympathetic and parasympathetic systems.

The objective for athletes is to introduce the right amount of physical and mental stress and then use the most efficient and effective form of adaptation. When athletes are not in a game or event, in a training session, or working up a mental sweat, they should be adapting through rest and refueling.

Adaptation is the process of becoming better suited to the environment, meaning improving. Simple breathing methods allow us to shift into a parasympathetic state, which fosters adaptation. These include extending the length of an exhalation, gently pausing after inhalation and exhalation, and creating a rhythmic breathing pattern. These examples emphasize slow breathing. Several complete breathing protocols will be covered in detail in chapter 8.

Nervous System Responses

Sympathetic Nervous System: Survival and Stress (Fight, Freeze, Flight)

The sympathetic nervous system is the body's built-in alarm system. In response to dangerous and stressful situations, the sympathetic nervous system floods the body with hormones to boost alertness and heart rate and to send extra blood to the muscles. The respiration rate also increases.

Responses to Sympathetic Activity

- Dilated pupils and a decrease in peripheral vision
- Inhibited salivation
- Constricted blood vessels
- Stimulation of glucose release and glycogen breakdown
- Increased heart rate and respiration
- Disrupted activity in the stomach
- Release adrenaline
- Loss of fine motor skills

Responses to Chronic Sympathetic Activity

- Performance anxiety, worry, and fear
- Fatigue and reactive emotions
- Irritability
- Sleeping disorders
- Hyperventilating and fatigue
- Cognitive dysfunction and tension in nonworking muscles

Parasympathetic Nervous System: Adaptation (Rest and Digest)

The parasympathetic nervous system regulates the body's ability to adapt. It is more engaged when we are in a relaxed state such as sleeping and eating. The following are responses to engagement of the parasympathetic nervous system.

- Constriction of pupils for a wider view with a relaxed gaze
- Stimulation of salivation
- Preparation for digestion by stimulating the intestines and contracting the bladder
- Slower heart rate
- Increased vasodilation to most organs
- Improved cognitive function and data assimilation
- Tissue regeneration and muscle growth
- Improved fine motor skills
- Relaxation, calmness, clarity, and creativity

Controlling Stress to Enhance Adaptation

Stress is necessary for developing higher functions such as overall well-being, mental acuity, and improved strength and endurance. In fact, we are the only species that can create an environment of controlled stressors in order to build strength—for example, the weight room, competitions on the playing field, or practice of a skill. Although introducing stress is necessary for improvement, it must be the right kind of stress in the right amount, and it must be followed by a period of adaptation. Failing to recognize the signals the body sends to indicate inappropriate stress or an imbalance between stress and adaptation causes the body to break down. Today, many of us live in a fast-paced, overstimulated world, and without adequate adaptation, our minds and bodies will start to compensate. Compensation takes place when our mind or body needs to achieve a mindset or movement pattern that has not yet been established or is unavailable to us. This means at some point the level of stress was too high, either mentally or physically, for the athlete to adapt. For example, an athlete may compensate with a stimulant to ease their mind or compensate by moving poorly to complete a stressful movement. Over time, the negative effects of compensation and lack of adaptation build up and lead to injuries in the physical body and anxiousness in the mind. The inability to recognize modern stressors has led to a rise in mental health issues. As a modern society, we seem to be picking the wrong stress and overexposing ourselves to it. This not only affects athletic performance, but it also affects all aspects of life.

Remaining in a state of stress outside of training and competition often leads to overbreathing and mouth breathing, which use oxygen inefficiently. This results in insufficient adaptation and energy mismanagement. We must learn to recognize a state of heightened stress and its indicators: higher respiratory rates and mouth breathing, which should be reserved for training and competition. If we are not supposed to be stressing the system, then we should not feel stress. Sources of unwanted stress could be chronic mouth breathing, poor breathing mechanics, or lifestyle choices. Unwanted stress also comes from lack of sleep, poor nutrition, negative relationships, and worrying about things outside a person's control. Negative stress comes from anywhere, and peak performers are brilliantly able to choose when and how to add stress rather than living in it.

Breath work is a tool that allows us to consciously change respiration while sitting or lying down. By breathing slowly and bringing the heart rate down, we enter a zone of recovery. Because the lungs are innervated by both the parasympathetic and sympathetic nervous systems, altering the breath puts the body into a different state. High respiratory rates caused by stress promote a sympathetic state. This is the case when we are training, competing, or experiencing excessive stress. On the other hand, slow, paused, and rhythmic breathing promotes a parasympathetic state. By consciously changing respiration, we have the ability to enhance adaptation and use the breath to recover from stressors.

Shifting Between States of Stress and Adaptation

Breathing, which is the only aspect of the ANS that can be consciously controlled, is the key to shifting between states regulated by the sympathetic and parasympathetic nervous systems. The more effectively we use breathing to shift between the two states, the more control and greater the self-confidence we will have while making decisions under pressure.

When the body perceives danger, the sympathetic nervous system creates a state of fight or flight. This response is meant for short-term emergencies. When used appropriately, we're able to get things done and compete at high levels. On the other hand, a parasympathetic state inhibits the body from overworking. The state created by the parasympathetic nervous system is focused on restoring, relaxing, and healing the body. When used appropriately, we're able to achieve greater levels of adaptation. Whether the body triggers the sympathetic or the parasympathetic nervous system depends on the stimuli in the environment.

Athletes who know their bodies well are aware of their breathing. If you're just beginning to develop this awareness, ask yourself the following questions. In these moments, should you be stressing your system (sympathetic) or adapting your system (parasympathetic)?

Do you notice your heart beating faster while you are on the bus to a game or practice?

Do you notice that your jaw has dropped and your tongue is resting at the bottom of your mouth while you're sitting in class or studying film?

Have you been in front of a computer screen all day and noticed you are breathing into your upper chest?

Have you been sitting too long and your lower back starts to hurt?

Do you feel reactive and emotional for no reason?

Do you feel rushed to start your day or have trouble sleeping?

All of these scenarios occur outside of athletic performance. Answering *yes* to any of them indicates that you are experiencing stress when you should not be. If you feel your heart beating fast, your lower back starting to hurt, or a dry mouth, or you have trouble remembering things, chances are you're spending time in a sympathetic state outside of athletic performance. This means you are using excessive energy and will enter a performance in a less optimal state.

As you recognize the feeling of stress in your body and what's triggering it, you can always tap into your breathing. Daily breath practice helps you grow an attachment to both mind and body. As you become aware of your breathing throughout the day, you will gain a better understanding of your general well-being.

Upper Airway, Lungs, and Muscles of Respiration

Three major components comprise the structures involved in breathing: the upper airway, the lungs, and the muscles of respiration. In the world of breathing, these are known as the big three and are the focus of this section. The upper airway includes the nasal cavity, pharynx, and larynx, and the lower airway includes the trachea, primary bronchi, and lungs. Together, the upper and lower airways make up the respiratory tract. Three groups of muscles control breathing: diaphragm, intercostal muscles of the rib cage, and abdominal muscles. See figure 2.2.

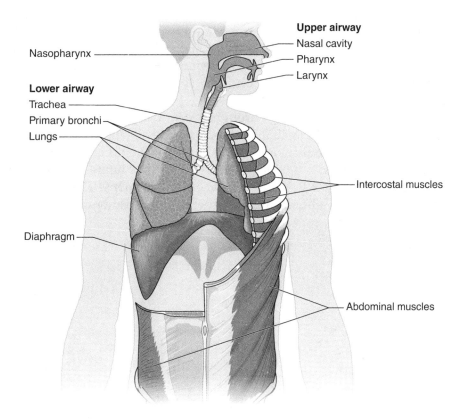

FIGURE 2.2   The respiratory tract and muscles of respiration.

Upper Airway

The nose is the gateway to the respiratory system. The nose has two nostrils that are separated by cartilage called the septum and can be felt on the front of the nose. Within the skull and surrounding the nose are air-filled cavities called the paranasal sinuses (see figure 2.3). These sinuses surround the nasal cavity and open into it to help the nose release nitric oxide. They are lined with cells that make mucus to keep the nose from drying out while we breathe. The nose warms the air as it enters the body to core body temperature. Inhaled air reaches 90 percent of the required temperature and humidity levels before reaching the nasopharynx (the top of the throat). The nasal cavity is the major conditioning apparatus in the respiratory tract (Zaidi et al. 2017).

The nose performs several functions that protect us. The olfactory bulbs, located at the top of the nasal cavity, receive useful neural input; for example, if food smells rotten we know not to eat it. Cilia, the tiny hairs on the surface of certain cells in the nose, provide feedback to the body and prevent illness. As they wave back and forth, they pull in odor molecules and send them to the brain for processing. The cilia aid in moving and eliminating dust, mucus, and bacteria from the body.

As air enters the nasal cavity through the nostrils, it meets by the turbinates, also called nasal concha. Turbinates are shell-shaped bony plates along the sides of the nasal cavities that cleanse, heat, and humidify the air as it travels through the nasal cavity on its way to the lungs. As air enters the nose, one nostril swells closed and the other one opens. This process is called the nasal cycle. The timing and intensity of airflow switching from

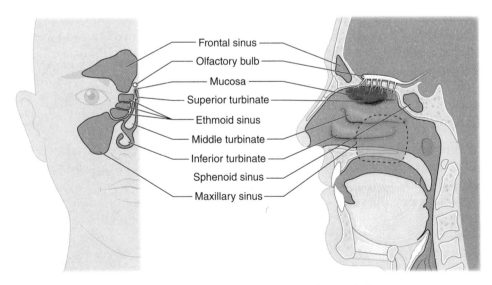

FIGURE 2.3   The paranasal sinuses, turbinates, mucosa, and olfactory bulb.

one nostril to the other varies from person to person. The nasal cycle keeps the mucous membranes in the nose from drying out. You may not notice this process taking place unless you have a cold or experience allergies.

Another unique function of the nose that helps keep us healthy is nitric oxide production. Nitric oxide is a molecule that helps us increase strength and fitness while decreasing recovery time. With each breath through the nose, nitric oxide follows the airflow into the lungs, and because it is a vasodilator, it helps open the airways and increase the oxygen uptake in the blood that feeds the muscles. This improves the gas exchange needed for respiration. Enzymes have been found in the nose, and specifically in the paranasal sinuses, that produce nitric oxide. This is the body's main site for nitric oxide production (Lundberg et al. 1995). Nitric oxide has many benefits:

- Increases health and elasticity of blood vessels
- Lowers cholesterol
- Relaxes smooth muscle as a vasodilator, which regulates and lowers blood pressure and improves circulation
- Works alongside carbon dioxide to assist with oxygen binding and release, which helps increase cellular oxygen uptake by 10 to 20 percent (see more in chapter 3)
- Controls vascular tone (regulation of blood pressure and distribution of blood flow between tissues and organs)

Another important benefit of nitric oxide is that it helps control our reaction to perceived dangers and stressors, and it reduces the effects of feeling afraid or nervous. This is why most of the recovery exercises in this book prescribe slow, calm breaths through the nose. The humming and hissing breathing protocols in chapter 8 accelerate the feeling of calm. Humming and hissing during exhalation can improve sinus ventilation as well as reduce stress, promote calmness, and lower heart rate and blood pressure. This happens because humming during exhalation exchanges the sinus gas and helps clear and calm the body more quickly than silent exhalation.

Lungs

When you think about breathing, you think of the lungs (see figure 2.4). The lungs are spongy, pyramid-shaped organs that sit in the chest cavity (thorax) next to the heart and above the diaphragm. They are attached to the trachea by the right and left bronchi. The major function of the lungs is to exchange oxygen and other gases from the atmosphere with the carbon dioxide in the blood. The air exchange that takes place in the lungs filters to the rest of the body thousands of times a day. Red blood cells then transport the oxygen from the lungs to other tissues in the body. This circulation is necessary to sustain life.

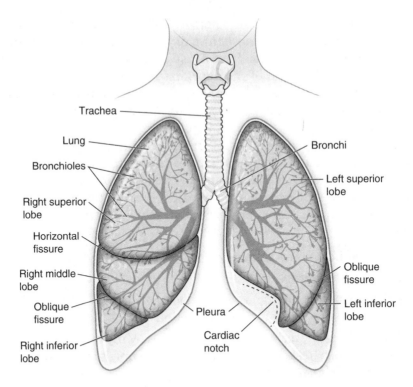

FIGURE 2.4   Anatomy of the lungs.

It is easy to think of the lungs like big balloons inside the chest cavity that inflate and deflate during the process of breathing. In certain breathing exercises, the balloon analogy can help you visualize the expansion of the ribs to create higher volume while inhaling. The lungs are covered with a pleura, a two-layered membrane that separates the lungs from the wall of the thoracic cavity in order to cushion and protect the lungs. The inner layer is the visceral pleura, and the outer layer is the parietal pleura. Visceral pleura wrap around the lungs and connect tightly. The close grip protects the walls of the lungs, keeping the organ intact. The thin space between the two layers of the pleura is the pleural cavity. It is filled with fluid that lubricates the cavity so the two layers can slide against each other without friction, which is essential to breathing.

Each lung is made up of lobes. The bigger and heavier right lung has three lobes—superior, middle, and inferior—separated by two fissures. The left lung, which is smaller and lighter, has two lobes—superior and inferior—and one fissure. Fissures are double folds of pleura that divide the lungs. The superior section of the left lobe has a middle area—the cardiac notch—that is unformed to allow room for the heart.

The lobes in each lung are supported by tubes called bronchi that begin at the bottom of the trachea and conduct air from the respiratory tract into the lungs and divide into bronchioles. The right main bronchus is wider

Cranial Nerves

The cranium is the skull, and cranial means toward the head or upper part of the body. Twelve cranial nerves connect the peripheral nervous system through the skull and into the rest of the body. These nerves support functions such as smell, sight, sensations in our face, and eye movement. The cranial nerves also help us balance, hear, and swallow.

The vagus nerve, which was discussed in chapter 1, is the longest cranial nerve. It wanders from the brain into the neck, chest, abdomen, and organs. How we breathe and stimulation of the vagus nerve are intertwined. During deep breathing, the vagus nerve gets less stimulation and promotes relaxation. Fast, shallow breathing stimulates the vagus nerve and triggers a fight-or-flight response. The vagus nerve sends communication from the brain to the gut. It is recognized for its role in the health of the mind and body because of its length and the stimulation of breathing.

To engage the parasympathetic nervous system you can take several actions to stimulate not only the vagus nerve but also all 12 of the cranial nerves. Splashing cold water on the face; massaging around the eyes, jaw, and cheeks; pulling your fingers across the forehead; and tapping your head all activate the cranial nerves. When deep breathing is coupled with stimulation to the face, the body relaxes and shifts into a parasympathetic state. Breathing exercises later in the book will outline ways to stimulate and use these nerves to improve health and performance.

and shorter than the left main bronchus. The right bronchus divides into three lobar bronchi, and the left divides into two. These lobar bronchi divide into tertiary bronchi (segmental bronchi) and are located within the bronchopulmonary segments of the lung. These functioning segments are split across each lung. Within these segments are alveoli, which are the tiny air sacs of the lung and are lined by an epithelium. The epithelium allows easy diffusion of oxygen and carbon dioxide and therefore a rapid exchange of gases between the capillaries and the alveoli. The tiny alveoli sacs sit at the end of bronchioles (tiny branches of air tubes in the lungs) like grapes at the end of stems. Think of the trachea as the main stem of a cluster of grapes, the smaller stems as the bronchi, the smallest stems as the bronchioles, and finally the grapes as the alveoli. The cluster of grapes represents the lungs.

You can think of alveoli as the smallest anatomical unit in the lungs. This is the site of gas diffusion between the lung and the bloodstream. The alveoli membrane is the surface of gas exchange from carbon-dioxide-rich blood pumped from the rest of the body into the alveolar blood vessels. Through the process of diffusion, it releases its carbon dioxide and absorbs oxygen. We have hundreds of millions of alveoli sacs in the lungs, and they are highly elastic. This allows the alveoli to stretch while they're being filled with oxygen during inhalation. Following this stretch, the sacs spring back during exhalation to expel air rich in carbon dioxide. Efficient gas exchange occurs when we take a full, deep breath.

Muscles of Respiration

The muscles of respiration expand the chest during inhalation and contract them during exhalation. Three groups of muscles control breathing: the diaphragm, the intercostal muscles of the rib cage, and the abdominal muscles. These muscles also contribute to safely performing natural movements in athletics. Natural human movements are squatting, lunging, pushing, pulling, bending, rotating, and gait (i.e., locomotion). If you cannot breathe while in any of these positions, you cannot move and perform properly.

Diaphragm

The process of breathing in and breathing out is dominated by the primary mover, the diaphragm (see figure 2.5). The diaphragm is a dome-shaped muscular and membranous structure that separates the thoracic cavity from the abdominal cavity. It spans from the front to the back of the body. It is the principal muscle in respiration and is anchored to the rib cage by a central tendon. The lungs cannot function without the help of the diaphragm. During inhalation, the diaphragm contracts and flattens, which enlarges the chest cavity. During exhalation, it relaxes and rises into the rib cage, pushing air out of the lungs. This process must take place to allow the exchange of all life force inside the body.

A simple difference in pressure occurs with each breath. Inhalation reduces the pressure inside the body to less than the pressure in the atmosphere so that air will rush in. To exhale, the diaphragm relaxes and returns to its dome shape, which make the thoracic cavity smaller, as shown in figure 2.5. As the thoracic cavity gets smaller on exhalation, it increases the internal pressure and forces the air out.

The cellular exchange and the effect of high altitude on breathing will be covered in later chapters, but for now think about hiking in the mountains. It is harder to breathe because the atmospheric pressure is lower at higher altitudes, which means you have to work harder to lower internal pressure.

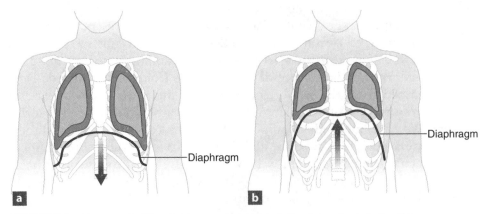

FIGURE 2.5   Movement of the diaphragm during inhalation (*a*) and exhalation (*b*).

We can build awareness of rib movement during breathing by recognizing that inhalation expands and lifts the rib cage, while exhaling contracts and lowers it. Being able to feel this movement and see it happening increases understanding of diaphragmatic breathing.

The respiratory muscles expand the rib cage, protect the spine, and align the hips and pelvis to move naturally. When we need to take in more air than usual, the diaphragm recruits help from the accessory breathing muscles—external intercostals, serratus anterior, sternocleidomastoid, and scalenes—to assist in lifting the ribs and expanding the chest. This is considered forced inhalation and exhalation because the breathing requires more force than normal. In the short term, we can recruit these additional muscles to assist in overbreathing, but these accessory muscles should not be the primary movers.

Accessory Muscles in the Cervical Spine Area

The cervical spine is located in the neck and consists of the first seven vertebrae. The accessory muscles in the neck aid in lifting and expanding the ribs during inhalation: the scalene muscles through their attachment to the first and second ribs and the sternocleidomastoid through its attachment to the sternum and clavicle. These muscles can be overworked with excessive breathing and breathing focused in the upper chest, and this can lead to chronic neck pain, nerve disruption, and fatigue.

The accessory muscles should be recruited only during intense exercises and competition. When accessory muscles are used for normal breathing, the diaphragm is not engaged, and breathing becomes shallow, which hinders proper oxygenation throughout the body. Tightness in the shoulders or neck and weak core strength are related to predominately using the accessory muscles for breathing.

Intercostal Muscles

Internal and external intercostal muscles lie between each rib and assist the diaphragm (see figure 2.6). During respiration, the intercostal muscles constantly work to move the rib cage. The internal intercostal muscles are deeper and depress the ribs to compress the thoracic cavity, which is a basic function of exhalation. The internal intercostal muscles help pull the rib cage down. The external intercostal muscles are used during inhalation. These external muscles work to elevate the ribs and expand the volume of the thoracic cavity. This allows the lungs to fill with oxygen. Although the external intercostals take part in the inhalation process, this book focuses on training and developing the diaphragm. This is because we can control the pace and movement of the diaphragm, especially during training and competition. While we don't consciously think about using our intercostal muscles during breathing, it's valuable to understand the role they play in breathing.

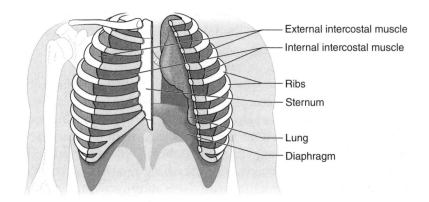

FIGURE 2.6   Intercostal muscles.

Figure 2.7 shows the relationship between breathing and the movement of the rib cage. Freely moving ribs create less stress in the breathing muscles.

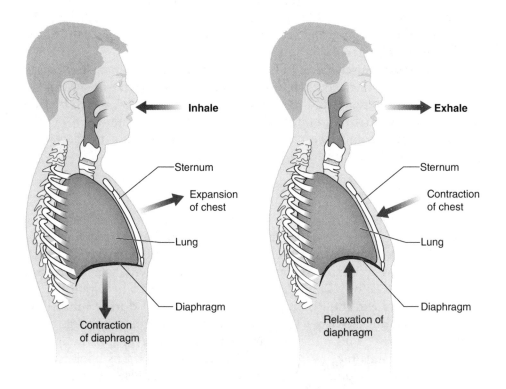

FIGURE 2.7   Movement of the rib cage during inhalation and exhalation.

Abdominal Muscles

The abdominal muscles pull the ribs down while breathing. Exhale forcefully while contracting your abs. You should be able to feel the ribs being pulled down as you're squeezing the muscles. During breathing, the external and internal obliques, rectus abdominis, and transversus abdominis muscles of the abdomen are engaged. These abdominal muscles are important during active expiration because they increase intra-abdominal pressure and force air out of the lungs.

Weightlifters work to develop intra-abdominal pressure (IAP) to brace the core during lifting. IAP should feel like having a safety belt around the waist. During inhalation, the diaphragm flattens and provides intra-abdominal pressure that causes the abdomen to expand outward. Because the diaphragm is attached to the lower ribs, this movement can be seen and felt as horizontal expansion. Take a deep breath in and try to fill the lungs with enough air to expand the entire belly and rib area. Try to feel the back of the ribs expanding. You should feel 360 degrees of movement in the ribs. Now hold that breath and feel the pressure around your body and spine. This is IAP and the pressure created through breathing. To feel this even more stand up and take a big inhalation. Feel the 360 degrees of rib movement, hold the air in, and perform a squat while holding your breath. Exhale once you have completed the squat. The breath should have created pressure to secure your spine, similar to wearing a weight belt.

Pelvic Floor

The pelvic floor is the lowest area of the body involved in respiration. The pelvic diaphragm (or pelvic floor musculature) is funnel shaped and controls the pressure beneath the organs and into the abdomen. While the thoracic diaphragm pushes down on inhalation, the pelvic floor moves with it. During exhalation, the pelvic floor pushes up against the organs while the thoracic diaphragm relaxes back into the rib cage. These two diaphragms maintain proper pressure and alignment of our internal organs.

The pelvic floor is made up of the levator ani muscles (largest component), coccygeus muscle, and fascia covering the muscles. These can be strengthened to improve hip mobility and protect the spine. It is important for athletes to feel these muscles and engage them through breathing, not only to keep the body healthy but to also build awareness as to what a full breath entails. To gain awareness of these muscles, take 10 breaths in through the nose and out through the mouth. On the exhalation, you should feel the muscles that you would use to keep from urinating. You should feel as if you're cupping your belly button in and up as the rectum is pulled into the body. This is the area between the anus and genitals. Exhalation pulls the pelvic floor muscles up, and you should be able to feel this during breath work.

The Bandha Locks

So far we have used a Western-based understanding of physiology and anatomy to explain the role of breathing to manage energy in the body. This is a relatively new perspective when compared to yoga practice, which has been around for thousands of years. Yoga is based on pranayama, which is the practice of breath regulation. In Sanskrit, *prana* means "vital life force," and *yana* means "to gain control." Bandha locks are used to close off specific areas of the body to direct energy where it is wanted. This is done by engaging certain muscles in combination with inhaling or exhaling.

The mula bandha, which refers to root, is engaged by lifting the muscles of the pelvic floor, specifically the levator ani, which is located around the perineum. This is the space between the anus and genitals. The reason for locking this root is to stop the escape of energy from the body. By using the mula bandha, you're able to stop the downward flow of movement. To feel the energy in this area, sit comfortably and breathe naturally. Contract the area and draw the muscles upward. Breathe fully for 4-5 breaths and relax.

The uddiyana bandha is the abdominal lock. It regulates the energy traveling up the center channel of the body. The lock sucks the diaphragm, abdomen, and stomach up and back. To engage this lock, sit comfortably and close your eyes. Take a deep inhale through the nose and exhale slowly all the air out through the mouth. Once all the air is out of the lungs, scoop the stomach in, contracting your abdominal muscles inward and upward. Hold here until you feel the sensation to breathe, gently release the stomach, and inhale gently through the nose.

The jalandhara bandha is the throat lock. To engage energy through this lock, inhale slowly and deeply. Draw the head forward while you lower your chin and press it down firmly into the collarbone notch. To enhance the experience, straighten your arms and press your palms to your knees to lift your shoulders. Hold this position for only a moment, then release the pressure of your hands on your knees and relax the shoulders. Exhale slowly and fully. It stimulates the vagus nerve, which controls the parasympathetic nervous system.

Through a Western lens, the muscles we engage to create the locks are the respiratory muscles. These include the diaphragm, rib cage muscles, and abdominal muscles as well as the muscles located at the base of the skull, in the neck, and in the upper chest. When doing breath work, it is important to understand these areas of the body, whether you're approaching it from an Eastern or Western perspective or incorporating ideas from both. The exercises in this book offer many breath practices that involve bandha locks. You can gain physiological benefits by pairing the two.

It may take time to feel the pelvic floor during breath work. Start by sitting with your body upright and the spine neutral by maintaining the natural curves. Take slow inhalations through the nose, feeling the thoracic diaphragm pushing down on the organs. Pause after the inhalation and then exhale through pursed lips. While exhaling, keep the spine neutral and notice the belly button slowly coming in toward the spine as you extend the breath. You should feel the area between the anus and genitals being contracted.

Understanding the role of the nervous system in breathing and understanding the relationship between the muscles responsible for breathing and the physiological processes of respiration form the foundation for establishing optimal breathing habits. The key to using breathing to drive improvement in athletic performance is recognizing stress as you are experiencing it and learning techniques to reduce it or adapt to it. You must be able to adapt so you can face the next challenge. As you spend more time with your breath and test it through the exercises in this book, your awareness will evolve, allowing you to master the stressors that lead to improved athletic performance.

3

Athletic Performance and the Breath

We manage energy through our breathing. This is because, in addition to what we eat, our body's ability to produce energy relies heavily on its ability to exchange oxygen and carbon dioxide. Each breath as we go through our day is important. This chapter describes the relationship between oxygen and carbon dioxide and the impact they have on athletic performance, how the body adapts to oxygen and carbon dioxide, and breathing principles that promote oxygenation for greater endurance.

Understanding How Oxygen and Carbon Dioxide Affect Athletic Performance

While breathing may seem like a simple process of bringing in air from the outside world into our internal world to maintain existence, the ability to use that oxygen to our benefit is trickier. At a basic level, breathing is inhaling oxygen into the lungs and then exhaling a waste product called carbon dioxide. Although carbon dioxide is considered a waste product and a toxic gas in the environment, it is crucial for breathing and plays numerous roles in the body. The carbon dioxide in the body is produced through tissue metabolism—the tissues use oxygen and form carbon dioxide. When carbon dioxide leaves the muscle tissue through the bloodstream, it is the catalyst necessary for the release of oxygen from the blood to the cells. These processes will be explored in this chapter.

Breathing is a complex process that relies on the coordination and action of the muscles of respiration (see chapter 2) and the control centers in the brain. The primary function of the lungs is to take in air to provide oxygen to the circulatory system and to remove carbon dioxide from the returning blood by exhaling it. Although carbon dioxide is considered a waste product, we need it to stimulate breathing and to optimize oxygenation. It does this by smoothing and widening the blood vessels as it leaves the tissues. This helps lower blood pressure, allows blood to flow into the extremities, and supplies oxygen to the brain and heart efficiently and effectively. This process keeps our nervous system from entering a stressed state, which allows healthy recovery and adaptation.

The second important role carbon dioxide plays in respiration is within the control centers of the brain. When we experience excessive carbon dioxide, the pulmonary system adapts and adjusts breathing patterns to meet the demands of the activity that caused the change in blood gasses. During training, oxygen consumption increases to provide fuel to working muscles, which raises carbon dioxide production. If we cannot take in enough oxygen to meet demand, carbon dioxide accumulates without disposal, the blood becomes acidic, and the cells of the body become damaged. To prevent this, the control centers signal us to breathe heavily through the mouth to aid in ridding the body of the excess carbon dioxide.

Consider the sensation you would feel if you were drowning or in need of air. These sensations are uncomfortable and stressful. You will experience some of these feelings during the breath-holding exercises in this book. These sensations occur when the body has built up too much carbon dioxide, and the brainstem interprets the feeling as "It's time to breathe now." Carbon dioxide controls the breathing rhythm at all times, which in turn controls the heart and brain rhythm.

To learn more about how oxygen and carbon dioxide affect performance, let's take a look at two key processes: energy production and the Bohr effect. These processes are a great starting point for deepening your understanding of how your body processes oxygen and carbon dioxide.

Aerobic and Anaerobic Energy Production

Oxygenating cells efficiently and effectively is important for athletic performance because cells need oxygen to produce energy through metabolism. To be a consistent performer and remain healthy, we must be a master at producing and maintaining energy. Sometimes we need fast-acting energy to finish a task and other times we need slow-burning energy to sustain us. Because breathing affects energy production, learning how to control the speed, depth, and consistency of the breath is crucial.

Metabolism is the chemical reaction in the cells that breaks down food into energy. When food is broken down to make fuel for the cells, the number one product of that breakdown is glucose. The chemical reaction in the cells when glucose is combined with oxygen produces carbon dioxide, water, and energy in the form of adenosine triphosphate (ATP). A simple analogy is to view yourself as a car and ATP as the gas that keeps it running. The body uses this fuel to produce muscle contractions and the power needed to move. Without this fuel your car would go nowhere.

ATP fuels the body in two ways: aerobically and anaerobically. Aerobic respiration is the most efficient form of metabolism and occurs when oxygen is available. This form of energy has enormous capacity, but it is unable to deliver energy quickly. In contrast, the other metabolic pathway, anaerobic respiration also turns glucose into ATP, but this time without oxygen. Anaerobic respiration creates bursts of energy, but because it is fueled only by glycogen, use of this precious fuel is reserved for intense exercise.

Ideally, we will spend more time using aerobic energy systems. This helps us sustain and control not only physical energy, but also mental and emotional energy. When an athlete is aerobically stable, they are able to fuel the muscles in the body with oxygen from the bloodstream without needing an additional energy source. When intensity increases and the athlete can no longer meet the energy demands of the muscles, the body uses its anaerobic system, which uses glucose stored in the body through a process called glycolysis. From an evolutionary perspective, if our ancestors needed to run from a lion, glycolysis was the precious fuel system that gave them the instant speed and energy to run away. Visualize controlled nasal breathing during a walk through the park and then erratic mouth breathing during sprints. If a lion is nearby, it is most likely you are not calmly nasal breathing but are mouth breathing as you sprint away.

We use anaerobic energy and heavy mouth breathing for intense activity that requires speed and power. When the demand for energy is low, we use the aerobic system. Mouth breathing is used to quickly take oxygen in and move carbon dioxide out. When muscles produce speed and power, the tissues metabolize and build up carbon dioxide in the body more quickly. Our natural reaction is to rapidly breathe through the mouth and off-load excessive carbon dioxide. However, removing carbon dioxide from the body quickly means less oxygen is delivered to muscle tissue because we need carbon dioxide to help release oxygen from hemoglobin. This book uses examples and provides ways to train athletes to perform nasal breathing to the best of their ability to maintain lower respiration and maximize oxygen consumption.

It is important to be aware of how you are breathing at all times. If you don't need to run from a lion, there is no need to breathe through the mouth or overbreathe. Controlled nasal breathing should be used in daily activities and during low-level aerobic activity. This will take an extended period of time adapting to this practice, but let your breath govern the effort. To help build consistency, you should also breathe slowly and through the nose while warming up for heavy training or competition. This will help keep a low respiration rate as well as engage the diaphragm fully.

While most coaches recommend breathing through the nose and mouth during training and competition, this book has a unique focus of developing the ability to breathe through the nose for as long as possible while exerting energy. This not only helps an athlete stay aware of their breathing, but trains them to breathe slower as long as possible. The mouth is used for larger volumes of air in and out and most certainly needs to be used at times in training and competition. Nasal breathing, however, keeps the respiration rate lower, and the value in keeping a low breathing rate is touched on throughout this book. By focusing on nasal-only breathing during low-intensity activities, you will fuel your muscles with oxygen more effectively with the lower respiration rate. It will also keep your nervous system in a relaxed state, free from perceiving a threat.

For example, during a long-distance run, it is best to maintain a consistent flow of light breathing for as long as possible and, more often than not, this means to focus on controlled nasal breathing. This is because long-distance running is an aerobic activity. As the runner gets to the end of the run, they may start breathing heavier and through the mouth, but the goal is to hold off from heavy mouth breathing for as long as possible. On the other hand, a sprinter running 100 meters will exhaust all energy as quick as possible and will not be as concerned with controlling their focus and attention in such a short amount of time. Sprinters, you will notice, breathe through their mouths right away because a short burst of energy is needed to meet the demand of the sprint. In this scenario, breathing at a lower rate is not a top priority for the sprinter.

To improve high-intensity performance and use reserved energy appropriately, you must begin with low-intensity activities to maximize your aerobic capacity. You can then begin adding anaerobic work to delay the point at which you experience fatigue. As you build a base and aerobic capacity with controlled slower breathing, you establish a bigger motor and a higher threshold to withstand the stress and demands of training and competition. With a bigger motor, you are able to sustain energy levels longer.

Using the Gear System

As children we were told the story of the race between the tortoise and the hare. The hare quickly gains a big lead and is so confident he will win that he takes a nap. The tortoise, although moving slowly, never stops and wins the race. The moral of the story is that you will be more successful by proceeding slowly and steadily than carelessly and quickly.

Brian Mackenzie, a human performance specialist and cocreator of the Art of Breath, an education clinic for breath work, uses the fable to explain the value of and differences between aerobic and anaerobic energy. The hare may go fast, but he can't go far, while the tortoise may not go fast, but can go far. We use aerobic energy like the tortoise does to be able to go far and last longer, and we use anaerobic energy like the hare does to move powerfully and quickly. As athletes, we are able to choose which animal to be. When we breathe through our nose, we act like the tortoise, using aerobic energy and activating the parasympathetic nervous system while keeping a low heart rate. When we breathe through the mouth, we act like the hare, using anaerobic energy and activating the sympathetic nervous system to create a fight-or-flight response and a higher heart rate.

In athletics there are times and places to be the hare—moving fast and burning energy—such as intense training, the end of a training session, or in a sprint. On the flip side, there are times to move slowly and burn less energy while acting more like the tortoise. Compare a starting pitcher in baseball to a closing pitcher. The starter is expected to pitch many innings and go deep into games, while a closer is expected to throw only one or two innings. While a starting pitcher wants to sustain energy and not tire too quickly, a closing pitcher is not concerned with conserving energy. One pitcher must maintain controlled breathing longer, which is the starter. They need to be aware of when it is time to be the tortoise and when it is time to be the hare. This may mean they need to gear down in between innings and focus on slowing down their breathing or pay attention to slow nasal breathing only. The closer may not be as concerned with being a tortoise or the need to control the pace of their breathing because they are only competing for such a short time. This is similar to the example of different expectations for energy use in a long-distance runner versus a 100-meter sprinter. Energy use is different depending on the individual, the position, and the sport.

Mackenzie and Rob Wilson, who cocreated the Art of Breath with Mackenzie, developed a five-gear system to help athletes determine when they should conserve energy and when they should use it—or in other words, when they should be the tortoise and when they should be the hare. Many times athletes try to force nasal breathing, which causes extra stress on the body and is counterproductive. The gear system is a guide to help athletes understand the energy they're using and the breathing demands for a specific task. Chapter 9 uses a gear system similar to this while training in cold exposure. Here, the five-gear system is meant to help an athlete understand the energy demands of nasal breathing versus mouth breathing:

Gear 1—Nasal inhale/nasal exhale

Gear 2—Power nasal inhale/nasal exhale

Gear 3—Power nasal inhale/power nasal exhale

Gear 4—Nasal inhale/mouth exhale

Gear 5—Mouth inhale/mouth exhale

The Bohr Effect

In 1904, Danish physician Christian Bohr discovered that carbon dioxide facilitates the release of oxygen from the blood to the cells. Oxygen is carried through the body by the hemoglobin, which exists inside the red blood cells. If carbon dioxide levels in the blood are low enough, oxygen and hemoglobin stay bound together, and muscle tissue will not receive the oxygen from the blood. Bohr discovered that carbon dioxide is the catalyst causing hemoglobin to release its grip on oxygen and supply it to the tissues. He realized that the more carbon dioxide in the body, the more efficiently oxygen is delivered.

Athletes who use breath practices to better use oxygen in the body should understand the Bohr effect. The longer an athlete can sustain a lower respiration rate, the better they handle buildup of carbon dioxide. At some point in performance, an athlete will feel out of breath or panicked. Blood oxygen levels are not the issue; instead, what is making the athlete feel like they can't get enough air is their ability to deliver oxygen into the cells. They are most likely hyperventilating and overbreathing, thus off-loading too much carbon dioxide.

The Bohr effect causes the muscles and tissues to release more oxygen when carbon dioxide levels rise. It helps deliver oxygen to metabolizing tissue such as skeletal muscle, where it is needed most. If the muscles are not oxygenated, they cannot work. If the muscles can't work, neither can the athlete. By breathing more slowly and training the mind and body to tolerate carbon dioxide buildup during times of stress and intense movement, the athlete will maintain oxygenation throughout the body longer. The Bohr effect is important because as carbon dioxide increases in those muscles of respiration, oxygen delivery to those muscles also increases. This helps the athlete continue to push through strenuous activity and continue to exert energy with a lower respiration rate.

Maximizing Carbon Dioxide Tolerance

As you move your body, the production of ATP (which is needed for movement) creates carbon dioxide. Carbon dioxide levels start to rise and eventually reach a point where the body needs to get rid of it. This point is your carbon dioxide tolerance, or carbon dioxide sensitivity. If you have a low carbon dioxide tolerance, you have to breathe harder and faster at low levels of intensity, making it more difficult for the cellular exchange to off-load oxygen into the muscles that need it most. You will experience more moments of breathlessness and reach exhaustion more quickly. The good news is that you can improve your carbon dioxide tolerance and raise your baseline, which will boost performance. To improve this tolerance, you should incorporate nasal-only breathing into your training, learn how to fluidly move in sync with your breath, and engage in regular breath holding, both in and outside of performance. Here are a few of the benefits associated with controlled breathing and incorporating breath-hold techniques into your training:

- Increases carbon dioxide tolerance so the body can handle rising carbon dioxide levels during physical exertion so you will naturally breathe more slowly.
- Increases aerobic endurance (creates a bigger motor).
- Oxygenates cells more efficiently, leading to less strain on the respiratory and cardiovascular systems.
- Manages energy.

Breathing Through the Nose

Nasal breathing allows us to breathe more slowly while actively using the diaphragm. This is the optimal way to breathe. Consistent nasal breathing automatically keeps carbon dioxide in the body, allowing us to more efficiently supply oxygen to the muscle tissue and maintain a state of balance. Over time, as we focus on nasal breathing, we increase our tolerance to the carbon dioxide buildup, which improves athletic performance.

Forcing yourself to change your breathing can be difficult at first. Allow yourself to enter this space with a beginner's mindset, and keep the end goal in mind: breathing entirely through the nose during rest and recovery. And then, outside of necessities like eating and talking, reserve mouth breathing for intense training and competition. You are trying to train yourself to breathe slowly through the nose to control your breathing during stress, which will translate to optimal performance in competition. For example, in yoga, a major principle is being able to control the breath while holding a difficult position for an extended time. To do this, you need to slow your breathing and find comfort in an uncomfortable position. As you train yourself to breathe through your nose, you might feel like you're going backward. Making progress requires a great deal of intention and focus. You might need to slow your workouts or decrease sets and reps. Your body will adapt, and you will be able to train at the level you are used to, except this time you will be breathing through your nose only.

As you increase the intensity of the exercise and begin to heavily mouth breathe, you will start to overbreathe. Your heart rate rises quickly and you are not able to supply enough oxygen to the muscle tissue to meet the demands, so you enter an anaerobic state and your source of energy is limited. The goal of this book is to teach you how to breathe through your nose longer during physical training. You will also learn how to calm the nervous system during significant periods of intense exercise and mouth breathing and how to pair your breath with your movement to maximize oxygen consumption. Improving these systems allows you to go harder in your training while also going longer. This translates to both mental and physical confidence in competition.

Here are a few ways to keep the body in a balanced state throughout the day and create consistency in nasal-only breathing. You should build habits that support focused nasal breathing so you recognize the mental and physical feelings associated with a balanced state.

- The simplest and most effective way to begin building a tolerance to consistent nasal breathing is to stop breathing through your mouth except during eating, talking, and intense activity.
- Breathe through the nose during sleep and recovery periods in and out of training. Focus on resuming nasal-only breathing after intense exercise; when going into another event; and during intermissions, halftime, or delays in your game or event.

- Practice lowering respiration by taking your breath rate to five or six breaths per minute, all through the nose. Do this for 10 to 60 minutes each morning or night.
- Train the mind and body to eventually complete an entire workout through the nose. Start during low-level aerobic activities such as walking, light cycling, or light jogging.
- Wear mouth tape during the day and night as your body adapts to constant nasal breathing. This could be while you're working, reading, writing, or watching television.

Pairing Movement With the Breath

Proper movement as we breathe keeps oxygen filtering through the body and supplying the cells and tissue with energy. To breathe fluidly while moving in sport is a long-standing practice in the human performance field. Inefficient breathing can result in muscular imbalance, motor skill alterations, and physiological adaptations that hurt athletic performance.

A 2014 study showed a direct correlation between breathing pattern disorders and movement dysfunction (Bradley and Esformes 2014). The study used the Functional Movement Screening to accurately predict injury in individuals who demonstrated poor movement patterns. Subjects who scored poorly on the test showed breathing disorder patterns while exhibiting poor biochemical and biomechanical breathing. In many cases, athletes are not aware that their breathing is disordered, which increases their risk of poor movement patterns.

As discussed in chapter 2, proper biomechanics during breathing creates horizontal movement of the rib cage instead of vertical movement. The following exercise can help you recognize positive diaphragmatic movement and proper mechanics. Stand or sit tall and place both your hands at the side of your rib cage (see figure 3.1). Breathing entirely through the nose, inhale so that you feel the bottom ribs expanding laterally, or horizontally, into the palms and fingers. On each exhalation, the ribs should move back inward as the diaphragm falls into place under the rib cage. As you breathe, keep the tongue at the roof of the mouth and relax the jaw. For immediate feedback, do this in front of a mirror.

The benefit of lateral, or horizontal, breathing, especially during movement, is to protect the spine and promote healthy posture. Weak breathing muscles lead to declines in performance and greater risk of injury. This happens because when the spine is not protected by the movement of the diaphragm, the body compensates, which results in poor postures (i.e., rounded shoulders; forward neck; tight upper-torso, back, and neck muscles). It is not difficult to imagine how a collapsed body posture affects our breathing and overall performance.

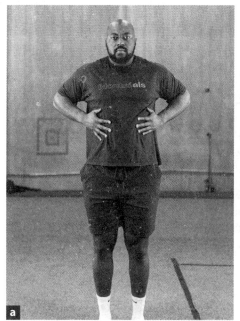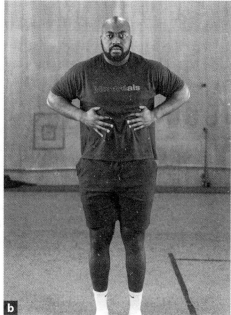

FIGURE 3.1 Exercise to learn the breathing mechanics for proper diaphragmatic movement: Inhale and feel the bottom ribs expand laterally (*a*); exhale and feel the ribs move back inward (*b*).

Breathing in Low-Oxygen Environments

When it comes to performance, forcing yourself into low-oxygen environments like high altitude to increase endurance offers many benefits. This type of training, called hypoxic training, referring to low levels of oxygen in the bloodstream (hypoxemia), has been commonplace at the Olympic level for many years. A trio of researchers—Dr. Gregg Semenza from Johns Hopkins School of Medicine, Dr. William Kaelin from the Dana-Farber Cancer Institute and Harvard Medical School, and Sir Peter Ratcliffe from Oxford University and the Francis Crick Institute—received the 2019 Nobel Prize in Physiology or Medicine for determining how cells sense and adapt to oxygen variations. In a nutshell, low oxygen levels in the body cause more of the hormone erythropoietin (EPO) to be produced in the kidneys, and because EPO controls the production of red blood cells, the low-oxygen environment stimulates the body to adapt by producing more oxygen-carrying red blood cells. The more red blood cells there are, the more oxygen can be delivered to working muscles, and the more oxygen that working muscles receive, the longer an athlete can work at a higher intensity without tiring out—hence the advantages of hypoxic training.

The Famous Wim Hof Method

The Wim Hof method, named for the Dutch extreme athlete, is a breathing practice that replicates controlled hyperventilation followed by holding the breath. Oxygen saturation rises to 100 percent while overbreathing, followed by a dip in the saturation levels during the exhalation hold. An athlete may find they can hold their breath much longer while doing this than they can with regular breath holding. That's because the hold releases carbon dioxide so quickly that the chemoreceptors can't pick up on the need to breathe.

Wim Hof popularized this breathing practice by displaying his tolerance for extreme cold and high altitude. Hof is known for climbing Mount Everest in nothing but shorts. In 2015, he and a group of amateur trekkers climbed the 19,341-foot (5,895 meters) mountain and set the Guinness World Record for a group. He also holds the Guinness World Record for sitting in an ice bath for one hour, 52 minutes and 42 seconds. Hof attributes this remarkable endurance and ability to how he breathes.

Functional magnetic resonance imaging (fMRI) analyses back up his claim, indicating that the Wim Hof method activates primary control centers for transcending pain or cold stimuli. By breathing deeply, Hof is able to make the blood more alkaline, which briefly turns off pain receptors in the brainstem, enabling him to withstand the shock of sudden cold temperatures.

This technique is safe for anyone who doesn't have underlying health issues and as long as they are not in water or driving. Breath holding following hyperventilation may cause a person to feel lightheaded or like they will pass out. If this occurs, they should focus on breathing slowly and rhythmically through their nose. Directions for hyperventilative breathing practices are provided in part II. People report that after a few rounds of breathing similar to the Wim Hof method, they experience a composed adrenaline. If the breathing practice brings about clarity, focus, and control, it is working. If it brings anxiety, panic, and worry, it is not.

Many studies have shown the positive training effects of a low-oxygen environment. However, we don't need to travel to high altitude to reap these benefits. Dr. Luciano Bernardi, an Italian professor of cardiology, found that a group of professional mountain climbers who practiced breathing at six breaths per minute for one hour daily for two years before attempting to climb Mount Everest were able to better use oxygen during their ascent (Bernardi et al. 2006). By training to take fewer breaths per minute, the climbers improved their ability to handle low-oxygen environments. The climbers in the study reached the summit without auxiliary oxygen and with a respiratory rate of only 10 breaths per minute. A control group of professional climbers did not practice breathing and needed to use oxygen tanks and struggled to breathe at the peak. One main difference between the groups was their breathing rate. The group that reached the summit took far fewer breaths.

Dr. Bernardi discovered that the climbers who practiced breathing were able to use 80 percent of the surface area of their lungs compared to the 20 percent typically accessed by most athletes. Dr. Bernardi also found that a respiratory rate of six breaths per minute caused the capillaries in the hands and feet to dilate, resulting in maximal blood flow to the extremities (Brown et al. 2012). This could offer an important advantage to athletes who rely on their arms and legs in competition.

Decreasing the number of breaths per minute is one method of breath holding, or creating a lower-oxygen environment. Other ways to simulate low-oxygen environments will be explored in chapters 5 and 6, but for now all you need to know is that when you're practicing breath holding for low oxygen, you hold the breath after the exhalation. When you exhale, you decrease the amount of air in the lungs, which causes carbon dioxide to build up faster. This buildup can feel uncomfortable and scary when the chemoreceptors in your brain react to low levels of oxygen and high levels of carbon dioxide in your blood by telling your brain it's time to breathe. The lower the level of oxygen and higher the level of carbon dioxide, the more urgent those signals become. Therefore, start these exercises slowly. Training yourself to manage low-oxygen situations through slow-paced breathing and breath holding can reduce the sensitivity of chemoreceptors to hypoxia (too little oxygen) and hypercapnia (too much carbon dioxide), which will lessen the panic reaction.

The following are benefits of breath-holding and low-oxygen practices. This will help you understand what takes place when you hold your breath.

- Increases carbon dioxide tolerance, which increase aerobic endurance.
- Increases nitric oxide, which dilates the blood vessels and opens the nasal pathways.
- Increases the strength of the diaphragm. Breath holding forces the diaphragm to contract, and over time this strengthens the muscle, which improves its function during performance.
- Increases red blood cells, which improves the oxygenation of the cells and muscle tissue.
- Increases mental resiliency and focus.

Patrick McKeown, author of *The Oxygen Advantage* and *The Breathing Cure*, often uses breath holding, specifically exhalation breath holds, with his athletes to improve athletic performance. In conversation with Dr. McKeown, he says that through breath holding, "We're deliberately inducing a state of breathlessness, far beyond what you would experience during high-intensity interval training. We may be training the brain. We may be resetting the central governor. We're telling the body you can push yourself harder and faster without overdoing it." McKeown states that forced breathlessness in training "opens up the airways, opens up the nose, opens up the bronchioles to the lungs. We also increase blood flow to the brain and an extra load to the breathing muscles." He also says that few people are doing this in their training, but the ones who are will reap the benefits (personal communication).

Take a second to put the book down and take a normal breath. Following the exhalation, hold your breath until you feel an urgent need to breathe. When that happens, follow the hold with a controlled inhalation. Don't worry about the length of your breath hold; instead focus on controlling your response. The more you practice this, the more you'll improve your ability to override the stress messengers in your body. Not only will breath-hold training improve your physiological endurance, but it will also strengthen your mental resiliency.

The goal of this chapter is to build a stronger understanding of how breath affects energy, which affects athletic performance. Achieving the long-term benefits of proper breathing takes consistent practice over time. If it is difficult to find time for dedicated practice, use moments here and there during the day to focus on nasal-only breathing: when you're warming up for training or competition or even just walking around town. Pause to become aware of your breath and make sure you're breathing through the nose. These moments throughout the day offer opportunities to maximize each breath. At the same time, concentrate on pairing your breathing with your movements. Eventually this will happen without your having to think about it, and you will feel connected with your breathing while being in the moment of movement. Finally, build a tolerance to carbon dioxide and strengthen the body's nervous system through breath-holding exercises. Many practices in this book involve breath holding. It is important to become comfortable with the sensations this causes, so you can make breath holding a part of your routine and benefit from the adaptations this training supports. Over time you will learn the depths of your gas tank and know when it is time to be the tortoise and when it's time to be the hare.

4

Emotions and the Breath

Most athletes would agree that to reach and sustain peak performance, they must be in control of their emotions. Emotional intelligence is a person's ability to understand, use, and manage their own emotions so they can control themselves in positive ways to relieve stress, communicate effectively, overcome challenges, and empathize with others. Athletes with high emotional intelligence understand their bodies and connect with their breathing to have a better awareness of what their emotions tell them. An athlete's ability to manage their emotions while also understanding the emotions of those around them results in greater self-awareness and self-control. It also makes them better teammates and communicators and better equipped to make decisions in the heat of the moment. Creating positive breathing patterns to help keep the mind and body sharp is key to achieving emotional balance. In this chapter, you will learn how closely connected the breath is with thoughts and emotions. Through this understanding, you can use the power of breath to overcome irrational emotions and negative thinking.

Breathing and Its Effect on Emotion

On average, we take 20,000 breaths a day, and that number could be as high as 25,000 or as low as 15,000. The point is, we take a lot of breaths each day. The majority take place when we are not training or competing, and chronic overbreathing or mouth breathing can significantly increase the number of breaths we take in a day. The theme throughout this book is to learn to breathe more effectively and efficiently so we can breathe more slowly during our day-to-day life. In previous chapters, we learned that a higher respiration rate, especially through the mouth, can engage the sympathetic nervous system and initiate fight-or-flight activity. We are not able to think logically when our breathing is chronically rapid, thus impairing performance. So this chapter continues to support the principle of slowing respirations and breathing through the nose.

When the body is in homeostasis and breathing slowly, the mind is calm. When the body is off balance, the mind will default to negative thinking and unregulated emotions. In sport, this is displayed through emotional reactivity, meltdowns, and frustration. These poor behaviors affect athletic performance and affect the longevity of an athletic career. This chapter outlines how breathing affects the mind and emotions and evolutionary principles that affect memories and have allowed the human species to survive.

For the majority of humans' time on Earth, our fear-based brain needed to protect us from harm. And we needed our senses to guide us through life. If it smells rotten, don't eat it. If it sounds alarming, run. It is likely that responses to these stimuli caused faster breathing through the mouth, and this change meant danger was around. Although today most of us have safe sources of food and we aren't likely to face lions, we still experience these changes in our breathing. Today it's more likely that anxiety is caused by worrying about what our peers think of us, the news we take in, or the status of our jobs. Humans overbreathe not only because of our recently weak jaws and sedentary lifestyle, but also because of the constant stimulation we receive.

In addition, the modern lifestyle can contribute to poor breathing habits. As discussed in chapter 1, chronic mouth breathing and upper-chest breathing activate the sympathetic nervous system. A chronically aroused sympathetic nervous system keeps us in a state of anxiety and stress. Constant stress decreases the time between stimulus and our response to it, often leading to inappropriate reactions (we'll talk more about this later in the chapter). Stress leads to emotional imbalances through negative thoughts and self-talk, which keeps us in a state of fear, anxiety, depression, pain, or other negative states. Our thoughts and self-talk heavily influence these experiences; therefore, chronic improper breathing patterns that keep our nervous system in a sympathetic state (fight or flight) need to be controlled and reversed in order to shift our perspective. Otherwise, we constantly feel as if we are running from a lion, which makes it extremely difficult to perform at a top level.

Many of today's mental skills training programs for sport focus primarily on our thoughts and how we make decisions based on our self-talk, how to control thoughts and emotions to reframe our attitudes and beliefs. Just as our ability to think positively can alter the biology of the body, so too can improper breathing make it difficult to reframe our attitudes and beliefs. Even though we can work to prepare our minds, when the pressure is on and the stress is high, our physical performance, cognitive control, and emotional intelligence is in the hands of respiration. We can succeed or self-destruct in the moment depending on how we breathe.

As you use the practices presented later in this book to balance emotions, remember that sports are exciting because no one knows the outcome of a contest. This makes it an experience of uncontrollable moments, creating in-game problems that only levelheaded and emotionally intelligent athletes can handle. As you become more confident in your breath, you are better equipped to manage your physiology, creating the psychological space to perform rationally under pressure. Your breath will create the psychological space between stimulus and your response to it to make rational decisions, as the space between the two expands.

Breathing and Its Impact on the Emotional Center of the Brain

Emotions are complex feelings that result in physical and psychological changes, influencing thought and behavior. Our emotions are the body's response to an interpretation of neurological, physiological, and cognitive experiences based on past experiences and through a release of hormones. This means that not just our thoughts but also our brain chemistry and physiological processes create emotion. While our thinking and behaviors may drive emotions, we can learn to use the breath to shift our nervous system so it aligns with the sorts of thoughts and behaviors we want, thus making our breath the focus of control in the emotional centers of the brain.

The limbic system is the part of the brain responsible for our emotions and behaviors. This region of the brain is located just above the brainstem and under the cerebral cortex. It is responsible for fulfilling many of our survival needs such as feeding, reproduction, caring for our young, and our fight-or-flight responses. Existing within the limbic system (see figure 4.1) are the thalamus and hypothalamus, which are responsible for our sense of thirst and hunger and for mood; the hippocampus, which is responsible for memories and learning; and the amygdala, which is responsible for our feelings of pleasure, fear, anxiety, and anger. The amygdala also attaches memory to our emotions.

Two major structures within the limbic system—the hippocampus and the amygdala—will play large roles in your ability to regulate and manage emotion based on fear and memories. The hippocampus is responsible for learning and holding memories. Think of the last time you went home for a home-cooked meal. The smell of your mother's cooking might have sparked an emotional response and a memory. This was the hippocampus being stimulated as the nose sent it sensory signals. The scent retrieved the memory

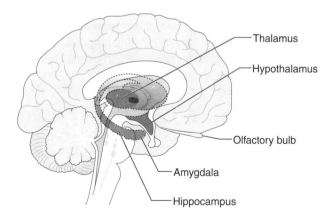

FIGURE 4.1   The limbic system of the brain.

The Triune Brain

In the 1960s, neuroscientist Paul MacLean formulated the triune brain model (see figure 4.2) that divided the human brain into these three categories:

- *Reptilian, or primal, brain*—responsible for homeostasis, arousal, and reproduction (governed by the basal ganglia)
- *Paleomammalian, or emotional, brain*—responsible for learning, memory, and emotion (governed by the limbic system)
- *Neomammalian, or rational, brain*—responsible for conscious thought, self-awareness, and verbal expression; doesn't fully develop until our mid-20s (governed by the neocortex)

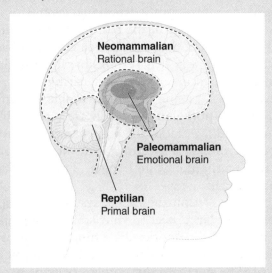

FIGURE 4.2   Triune brain model.

In MacLean's model, the reptilian, paleomammalian, and neomammalian parts of the human brain attempt to coexist. Recent research has rejected MacLean's model because newer imaging shows that multiple regions of the brain are active during primal, emotional, and rational experiences, meaning we can affect one layer of the brain by focusing on another. If we begin thinking of a memory that caused sadness, our limbic system activates an emotion. This can cause our breathing rate to increase, which elevates the heart rate. In this moment, our thoughts will change based on the emotion we're feeling and the way we're breathing. This is an example of the brain affecting all facets of the mind and body connection. MacLean's model may be outdated, but the triune brain model serves as a simple explanation of how the brain develops over time. We can use this model to better understand the workings of the human brain and where our impulse behavior stems from, how we experience emotion, and what area of our mind exists for self-awareness. Because we have conscious control over our breathing, we have the power to affect our emotions and thoughts while channeling energy and focus across the entire brain. The original MacLean model of the triune brain did not account for the connection between all areas of the brain.

of that food, and the emotion elicited by that memory was triggered by the amygdala. The amygdala is located next to the hippocampus and attaches emotions to our memories. Both of these centers in the limbic system are responsible for emotional responses.

The limbic system typically holds on to memories that are attached to strong emotional responses. Consequently, fearful experiences are formed and cemented into the limbic system more quickly than nonfearful experiences. When our senses take over and trigger autonomic responses, our breathing connects to the memories etched into our mind. For example, when we hear an unpleasant sound we've heard before that caused fear (or a similar sound), it triggers the amygdala to pull out a memory of that experience. In turn, our breathing rate increases and our heart rate spikes subconsciously and we begin to experience fear.

Recent research on how breath awareness regulates mood and emotion has focused on the limbic system. The Feinstein Institutes for Medical Research studied paced breathing to explore the effect of breathing on the brain. A specific style of breathing, here called paced breathing, uses neural networks beyond the brainstem to help regulate the response to stress. In the study, participants underwent brain scanning while they counted their breaths as they practiced fast- and slow-paced breathing to see how the brain responded to different breathing exercises. The study found that activity in the region of the amygdala suggests that a person's rapid breathing rate may trigger brain states like anxiety, or feeling states like anger or fear. Conversely, it may be possible to reduce fear and anxiety by slowing down the breath.

Training and competition naturally speed the breath, which activates the sympathetic nervous system. In performance, this is acceptable because an athlete wants to produce adrenaline and compete and train in an aroused state. However, it is equally important for an athlete to learn how to mentally and physically downshift from the acute sympathetic activity experienced in sport, and outside of performance focus their attention on slow breathing to reduce the sympathetic activity and resolve the fight-or-flight state. In the Feinstein Institutes study, participants were able to use the pace of their breathing to activate specific regions of the brain. In a performance realm, this means athletes can use breathing pace to manage their state of arousal. During training and competition, the breathing rate increases with the introduction of adrenaline, and athletes must be able to control this to be able to adapt and recover. One way is to practice slower breathing protocols outside of training and competition.

Our Connection to Smell

A study of the limbic system of rats found a nose–brain connection in the olfactory centers of these rats. Scientists found that the rats tied memory and emotion together based on smells. The stimulus of smell traveled through the olfactory system to reach the limbic system. Research has shown that humans also tie smells to emotion and memory. This is why the scent of clothes or a certain perfume can trigger a memory of a specific person, place, or moment in time. On the flip side, the smell of a food that caused illness can elicit feelings of disgust. This is the olfactory system sending signals to the limbic system, and whenever input reaches the limbic system, an emotional response can occur.

The olfactory bulbs, located in the forebrain, receive neural input and play a role in retrieving memories triggered by odors. It is believed that these bulbs are responsible for information processing in the brain. They sit at the top of the nasal cavity like wind chimes. When the sound of wind chimes becomes loud and hectic, we know the weather is changing. Wind, rain, and snow affect the flow of air through the wind chimes. The olfactory bulbs function similarly: When airflow brings scents or particles into the nose, the olfactory bulbs are stimulated and act like wind chimes sending signals to the limbic system and triggering an emotional response.

Breathing to Control Emotional States

Through inhalation and exhalation, your emotions are regulated by the way you breathe. When you are in a sympathetic state—anxious or fearful, for example—your breath is shallow and quick. When you're relaxed and content, your breathing is calm, slow, and deep. It's the slow, controlled breathing that takes place through the nose during the day that keeps you healthy. By maintaining slow, quiet, and rhythmic nose breathing, you are able to keep yourself in a parasympathetic state. This voluntary influence over your breath used in conjunction with training or in competition gives you an athletic edge. A simple technique to manage your breathing is to ask yourself throughout the day whether you feel like you're running from a lion. If you feel like your breathing is dysfunctional or you cannot control your emotions, chances are your nervous system feels like a lion is nearby. In sport, the only time you want the nervous system under stress is in training or competition. In all other aspects of life, there should be no lion.

Your perceptions and the subjective ways of seeing the world are learned from and influenced by your breath. You could say your breath is your teacher. The breathing practice that will allow you to control your nervous system starts with a slow, rhythmic breath. The exercises in part II offer a variety of ways to do this. For now, sit or lie comfortably in a supported position. Close your eyes and mouth, and breathe silently through the nose. Focus your attention on feeling the breath move in and out. As thoughts arise, bring your awareness back to the breath. Start with 5 to 10 minutes of slow, mindful breathing once or twice a day as you work your way up to 20 to 30 minutes. Slower breathing leads to parasympathetic dominance rather than a balance between sympathetic and parasympathetic states, which creates a sense of calm and alertness that is ideal for all activities throughout the day.

With a clock or stopwatch in front of you, follow the seconds as you breathe in and out. Take a five-second inhalation with a pause and follow that with a five-second exhalation with a pause. Do not worry about matching the seconds on the clock exactly; simply use it as a guide to keep your mind focused on the breath. This pace should result in five or six breaths per minute. Breathing this slowly opens the capillaries to optimize blood flow and oxygenation of the extremities. Younger athletes can breathe faster and reduce the time. They should follow their breath for as long as their natural attention span allows, typically two to five minutes. Athletes age 10 and under should take 10 breaths per minute and follow the clock for two to three seconds on both the inhalation and exhalation, with a pause between the inhalation and exhalation.

Controlling Arousal Levels and Flow State

When the ability to control emotion is poor, we may experience negative thoughts, negative self-talk, and negative emotions. It is likely that when we experience any of these, our arousal levels are heightened and out of tune. The optimal state of living, or flow, is when we're aligned with our mission, connected with our values, and rooted in the present. Flow is necessary for peak performance and is the ultimate freedom of self-expression. When we feel we're able to perform at our highest level without forcing extra effort, that is flow. When we find ourselves out of flow, we are stuck in a state of heightened arousal. Our breathing, if left unmanaged, can take us out of tune and disrupt flow, leading to unwanted arousal.

Arousal can be broken into two groups: hyper or hypo. Hyperarousal is a heightened state of anxiety that we experience when we perceive something as a threat. We are hyperaroused when we're worried, jittery, or fearful. We are able to experience this state of anxiety even if the threat is no longer present. This could happen when we are caught up thinking about a previous mistake made in competition or fear a future failure. Neither of these exist in the present, which means flow is disrupted. Hyperarousal leads to overbreathing, which can, in turn, lead to hyperventilation. Chronic states of hyperarousal can induce anxiety, panic attacks, and fatigue. Hypoarousal is a state of feeling emotionally numb or socially withdrawn. This state of arousal can be triggered by traumatic memories and specific negative emotions. Being hypoaroused can make us sad, depressed, or chronically fatigued. Chronic states of hypoarousal can cause us to underbreathe or hold our breath, leading to brain fog, memory loss, and sleep disruptions such as sleep apnea.

It is helpful to think of flow as a river running between two banks: hyperarousal and hypoarousal (see figure 4.3). Just as a deep and wide riverbed

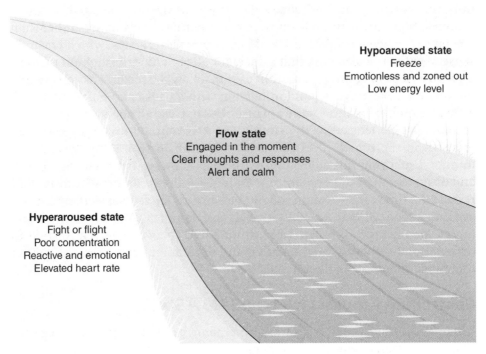

FIGURE 4.3   Flow state: the space between hypoarousal and hyperarousal.

allows water to flow smoothly without overflowing its banks, you can create space in your mind to support flow and decrease the likelihood of experiencing either a heightened aroused state or underaroused state for an extended time. This space in your mind gives you the freedom and power to choose your response to real-time stimulus and the pressure of sport. If the space in your mind is shallow or narrow, your reactions will be reactive and irrational, causing you to fold under pressure. Space in the mind sufficient for a sustainable flow state heightens self-awareness, improves critical thinking, and leads to emotional stability.

This book supplies the tools to widen and deepen the river of your mind. Slow, proper breathing coupled with a healthy lifestyle expand the space between the riverbanks, which is where your flow state exists. Flow is minimized by time spent in a hyper- or hypoaroused state. Training and competition slightly minimize the space because of the presence of adrenaline, but they do not pose a threat if you sustain calm, slow nasal breathing outside of them. You can use your breath to consciously shift the nervous system from creating a stressful environment to creating a safe and adaptive environment. When you are able to root yourself in the present, you are freed from assigning judgment. Creativity, imagination, and belief are accelerated when the chains are removed from the mind.

Overbreathing, mouth breathing, and upper-chest breathing lead to hyper- or hypoarousal that affects our emotions and thoughts. Because it can be difficult to recognize the trigger that took us out of our flow state, this book focuses on the breath as the center of control. It is often suggested to athletes that they get out of their mind and into their body when they feel they are not in flow. *Body* in this case refers to the breath. It is the one mechanism in the body that is rooted in the present that we can control.

Being unable to control the rhythm of breathing or chronically mouth breathing causes many cognitive processes to decline: memory, learning, language, and problem-solving. A 2021 study investigated the effect of oral breathing on cognitive activity using functional brain imaging (Jung and Kang 2021). The researchers confirmed a functional connection between working-memory tasks and breathing. The areas of the brain responsible for memory processing were less active when participants breathed through their mouths than when they breathed through their nose. This suggests that prolonged mouth breathing could impair cognitive function.

Success in training and competition requires pushing yourself until you must take in more oxygen by breathing faster and through your mouth. This stimulates the sympathetic nervous system, causing a heightened sense of arousal that allows you to think more clearly, run faster, and feel stronger. You cannot improve performance by staying in a balanced state dominated by the parasympathetic nervous system. The key to adaptation is to recognize the signs indicating that you have entered an aroused state and to know when and how to get out of it. During moments of flow, you may not notice physical signs, which is your mind's way of staying out of performance and allowing your body to perform freely. But when you notice your arousal level is too high, there are actions you can take.

Here are two questions to ask yourself when building awareness of unwanted arousal:

- Are your current emotions helping or hurting performance?
- Are you experiencing feelings or thoughts associated with hyper- or hypoarousal states?

If your answers indicate your emotions, feelings, or thoughts are hurting your performance, it is important to first identify the thinking patterns or feelings associated with the emotions and how often you experience them. Write out the thoughts or emotions and how often you experience them. Simply acknowledging the mental barriers that exist in your performance will begin to reduce their frequency. And writing them down will help you understand how your mind works.

After you acknowledge each mental barrier and either write it down or say it out loud, follow that with a cadenced breathing practice. First, acknowledge the mental barrier, then breathe slowly in through your nose and out through your nose at the same pace for three breaths. By becoming aware of the breath, you begin expanding the space in your mind to let irrational thoughts fade away as well as acknowledge that the anxiety is a past or future feeling, and then you can bring yourself back to the present. By becoming aware of the breath, you are able to center yourself and decide whether what you're thinking is in or out of your control. By realizing an event or experience is outside your control, you can let it pass and accept it for what it is. By realizing an event or experience is inside your control, you can develop the space in your mind to make the most rational and optimal decision. Once you feel you're in control again, unwanted anxieties and emotions should subside.

Understanding Negativity Bias and Emotional Triggers

Have you ever noticed that you dwell more often on the mistakes of performance than the successes? Criticism generally has a greater impact than praise. We commonly remember traumatic experiences rather than positive ones. We also react more strongly to a negative stimulus and think more often of negative outcomes than positive ones. Psychologists call this the negativity bias, and it is likely that this stems from our evolutionary processes of trying to avoid threat. Early in human history, paying attention to a threat and negative events was the difference between life and death. Humans who were more aware of the dangers around them or were capable of paying attention to the bad things nearby were more likely to survive (Cacioppo, Cacioppo, and Gollan 2014).

In athletics, failure to regulate emotions in response to bad calls, yelling from parents or fans, lineup changes, fatigue, and weather affect performance. When we process input improperly, our responses are dictated by emotional triggers that negatively affect our choices and behaviors. During these moments, our rapid breathing and heart rate and narrow field of vision provide warning signs that we are not thinking logically and are not able to make optimal choices. This is why asking an agitated person to calm down doesn't work and why a fatigued, highly aroused athlete will throw their helmet after striking out. While these emotional triggers have served an evolutionary purpose to protect us, today they don't serve as much purpose. Because we can't avoid situations our negative bias perceives as threats, we must become aware of their existence and learn how they trigger our emotions and their impact on our thinking and behavior. This knowledge gives us greater control over ourselves.

Our evolutionary processes and development of negativity bias have resulted in four major triggers, and even today, our natural response is to try to avoid them:

Uncertainty

Uncertainty in the form of fear of the unknown causes us to worry about a future event, and thinking about something can cause physiological responses in the body. As our mind races as we anticipate nerve-racking events, the uncertainty creates hormonal changes and increases the heart rate.

The initial news of COVID-19 placed the world in a state of uncertainty. We didn't know how to handle this new global virus. A few years after the initial shock, we have moved forward as a society to slowly resume normal activities, but these early stages of reintegration have caused anxiety. On a smaller scale, an athlete may experience anxiety because of uncertainty about the future of their career. Professional athletes are not guaranteed a next contract, and many high school athletes hope for a college scholarship. If this uncertainty about the future plagues the clarity of the present, it can hinder peak performance. "Anxiety is an emotional response to a perceived threat that's not actually there in front of you," says Mazen Kheirbek, PhD, associate professor of psychiatry and behavioral sciences at the University of California at San Francisco. Consider this statement the next time you feel your thoughts affecting you negatively.

Change

Change can also cause fear of the unknown and trigger avoidance behaviors. Again using COVID-19 as an example, dealing with the virus caused a great deal of change in how and where we worked or even if we were able to work, how we spent time with people, and how we managed all aspects of our health. This led to a great deal of anxiety.

For athletes, change is inevitable. Schedules, lineups, opponents, teammates, and coaches change. Most of the change that happens in sport is outside the athlete's control. This continued stimulus can lead athletes into emotional imbalances and anxiety. If they avoid dealing with the emotions caused by the change, the result will likely be poor performance. When facing uncertainty or change, it is crucial the athlete knows how to manage their emotions and adapt to the stress.

Attention

Competition in sport exposes athletes to attention, and as athletes progress through the levels to larger platforms, the attention increases. At the highest levels athletes deal with large fan bases, media outlets, and higher stakes, and attention can have a negative impact on performance. And even at beginner levels, attention has the potential to make athletes feel uncomfortable and overwhelmed as they fear rejection, loss of control, being ignored, or being criticized. When an athlete loses focus on the present and becomes consumed with the attention they perceive, they experience a heightened state of arousal. The sense of flow is eliminated, and the mind wanders away from peak performance.

Athletes early in their careers often are triggered by unaccustomed attention. An athlete who receives little attention doesn't feel the pressure of external expectations, and is able to perform successfully. However, once the athlete achieves enough success to gain attention, they can experience anxiety as they fear they will not be able to live up to the expectations of those around them or repeat their success. Before this anxiety, they were able to stay focused in the moment and perform in a state of flow. In this new state, their focus is on the attention they feel, which causes negative emotions that disrupt their flow.

Struggle

The difficulty presented by sport is also what makes the effort worth it. Athletes push themselves mentally, physically, and spiritually to try to reach the pinnacle of their sport. Yet their survival instincts lead them to find and secure comfort, which goes against embracing struggle. Anything that seems difficult induces some degree of fear because it's perceived as unsafe by their ancient brains.

We witness this in daily activities such as waking in the morning, working out, and speaking in public. These all require a level of struggle, and each time we decide against doing difficult things, we give in to our biological need to search for comfort. This is why we know self-discipline is more effective than motivation. As we discipline ourselves to push through a struggle, we not only continue to adapt, but we also become more confident in our ability to do hard things.

The negativity bias and emotional triggers are established through the perception of fear. These evolutionary responses were meant to keep us away from danger and to force us to find protection. Have you encountered a frustrated animal, spitting, clawing, or hissing at you? These animals are frightened, and they display defensive behaviors hoping you will leave them alone.

Similar to animals, it is in our nature to revert to a state of survival and flee from danger. When stressed, our pupils dilate, our heart rate increases, and our blood pressure rises as our breathing rate increases. These responses minimize emotional intelligence and limit higher cognition, hindering our ability to make rational and logical choices. Faster breathing triggers our mind to search through experiences we've tried to avoid and to use that for decision-making. Our breath becomes the language our thoughts will listen to. Many examples of this occur in sports. In baseball, for example, if a pitcher injures their elbow throwing a curveball and needs surgery to repair the torn ligament, their subconscious will keep them from performing movements that cause pain. After surgery, their subconscious will continue limiting their movements as they begin relearning how to throw a curveball. The thought of throwing a curveball and not knowing what could happen triggers physiological responses, hormonal changes, and respiratory changes.

Awareness of these four emotional triggers allows us to ask ourselves targeted questions to discover what has triggered us emotionally. Inevitably, we will face all four triggers during a career. The negativity bias comes into play and emotional imbalances occur during athletic performance when we perceive the route forward to be a threat and anxiety rises. The less able we are to regulate our level of arousal, stress, and emotions, the less likely we are to positively respond to negative stimulus. The arousal and stress experienced during athletic performance is managed through slow and controlled breathing. Mindful breathing that fully oxygenates tissue reroutes negative thoughts and creates a beneficial cognitive state and higher levels of awareness and perception. This allows us to assess feedback in the moment and make logical choices.

Managing Stress Through Emotional Intelligence

As athletes today, we are concerned with survival, and while our survival no longer relies on our ability to hunt and gather for food and avoid predators, we face emotional stressors our ancestors did not. A study in 2021 found that 4 in 10 adults in the United States reported experiencing anxiety or symptoms of depression. This number had increased from 1 in 10 a year earlier (Panchal et al. 2021). Athletes are not immune to this trend, so developing emotional intelligence is necessary for optimal performance. This requires us to prioritize where to spend emotional energy, which can be influenced by consistency in proper breathing and self-awareness.

The goal is to enter an athletic performance with maximized energy to handle the pressures and stress of being an athlete. After an activity that activates the sympathetic nervous system, we must focus on reaching a parasympathetic state and beginning the recovery process. Stress outside of performance that raises the respiration rate has a compounding negative effect on performance. This means that during the day, we must monitor our energy and emotional status and adjust our breathing as needed. Once training or competition has ended, we should perform a 10- to 15-minute down-regulating breathing practice to shift the mental and physiological processes of the body toward recovery. Recovery exercises and breathing protocols are listed in chapter 8.

It is unrealistic to ask an athlete to pay attention to all 20,000 breaths they take each day. A better route to optimal breathing is to minimize stress outside of training and performance. This includes breathing slowly through the nose during all adaptive periods of the day. It is also important to choose when to introduce stress to the mind and body and when to avoid it. These behaviors and thought processes will develop balance, control, and high emotional intelligence.

How breathing affects our nervous system was not well understood until neuroscientists and neurophysiologists began to find that the brain responds to breathing patterns. Further research has shown that our breath does more than just keep us alive, but also affects general well-being. Slow, controlled breathing influences the brain to produce optimal performance and flow. Slow nasal breathing throughout the day contributes to longevity and enhanced mood. Sustained nasal breathing also leads to brain health and cognitive processing between the limbic system and neocortex, which improves emotional intelligence.

When you become overly fatigued or begin to mouth breathe in response to a high-stress situation, your ability to think logically and make decisions is impaired. You may also experience a decrease in fine motor skills and endurance. Use mindful attention to breathing with intentional changes in the rhythm to manage the activity in the limbic system.

Breathing influences cognitive processes. And controlled breathing can encourage positive self-talk and positive feelings that help control emotions. Breath control, which has been shown to improve cognitive disorders through therapeutic work, can also improve cognitive processes during competition. By working on your breath outside of training and competition and learning to recognize stressors, your body will be better able to recognize and manage your reaction to them. This will improve your decision-making and performance in high-stress situations, and also increase the amount of stress you can experience before performance is impaired. A calm, rhythmic breathing cycle is necessary to manage the stressors inherent in a game, event, or competition and maintain control over the moment. Focusing on the breath improves cognitive responses to stimuli and supports appropriate emotions in the face of in-game pressure. Controlling your breath controls your emotions.

Part II
Breathing Exercises

5

Exercises to Test and Measure the Breath

Today we have access to a variety of biofeedback devices that measure physiological factors such as heart rate, muscle tension, and breathing patterns to help us understand how our bodies are functioning and reacting; however, it's important to recognize the cost this technology can have on our ability to tune in to our own bodies. As Laird Hamilton, a big wave surfer highly involved in breath work, says, "By being more connected, we become less connected" (2019). These are confusing times. We have more resources than ever before, yet athletes across the board are becoming weaker, more injury-prone, and experiencing performance anxiety and burnout.

Rather than inward reflection, feedback from watches, monitors, and tracking devices often leads our decisions about training. We feel that because we have this technology, we should use it to make choices instead of relying on how we feel. This makes it difficult to gain wisdom about our bodies, can cause us to lose confidence in ourselves, and makes it difficult to coach ourselves. Instead of using these tools alongside the knowledge we have about our own bodies, this technology can make it harder to know ourselves, and we pay the price in stagnant athletic advancement.

This chapter provides warm-up protocols to use before breath training and a variety of tests and measurements to help you understand your breathing. While breathing measurements can be subjective, these tests give you something objective you can focus on and improve. Adaptation and improvement can take weeks and even months to achieve. For this reason, it is important to establish the "why" behind breathing and to understand the value of long-term benefits rather than immediate justification. And, finally, keep in mind that breathing is an internal language you must learn, and this is a lifelong process. There is no end to your pursuit of better breathing. Regardless of where you're starting, keep it simple, focus on positive breathing mechanics, and remain aware of your breathing during the tests and the sensations that come with holding your breath.

Breathing Practice Principles

The following principles should guide your breathing practice and do not need to be followed in a specific order.

- *Take your time.* Because the adjustments that take place in breath control are small, set an intention to leave each breath practice with a heightened awareness of your breath, and take enough time to accomplish this.
- *Maintain a neutral spine.* Neutral does not mean straight. The spine has a natural S-shaped curve when viewed from the side: The cervical spine (neck) curves slightly inward, the thoracic spine (middle of the back) curves outward, and the lumbar spine (lower back) curves inward. Maintaining a neutral spine means maintaining these curves through the neck and back.
- *Avoid using the upper chest and neck muscles when breathing.* When you breathe into your upper chest and neck, you're most likely overbreathing and, more importantly, you are not accessing the diaphragm.
- *Focus on lateral movements at the bottom of the rib cage that promote horizontal breathing.* This will keep you from breathing into your upper chest and neck. It will also promote diaphragmatic breathing. This will help expand the rib cage 360 degrees and massage the organs below the diaphragm.
- *When nasal breathing, maintain a relaxed jaw.* Keep the tongue at the roof of the mouth and behind the top teeth. This will keep the airways open, and it makes it easier to breathe through the nose.

Breath Training Warm-Up Protocols

Before you perform a breathing exercise, warm up the face and neck. This includes the areas around the nose, forehead, eyes, jaw, lymph nodes, and voice box and key neck muscles. You can use these warm-up protocols to activate the nervous system and prepare it for breath work for any exercise in this book.

Nose Warm-Up

The nose is the primary structure for taking in air and letting air out. To start building effective nose breathing, wake the nose with a warm-up. It is common to experience a stuffy nose or suboptimal function in the nasal cavity when it isn't being used properly. This happens most often in the mornings after waking up, during extended time indoors, or in changes in climate due to temperature, humidity or the day's pollen count. When your nose functions poorly, take a seat and begin to wake it. This process can be used in mornings, before a training session, and before competition.

Nostril Warming

Rub your hands together until you feel heat in your palms (see figures *a-b*). Gently rub your hands on both sides of the nose. Start at the front of the nose, rub down the sides, and then rub between your eyebrows (see figures *c-d*). As you're rubbing your nose, breathe through the nose and extend the exhalation so it's twice as long as the inhalation. Focus on keeping the tongue at the roof of the mouth behind the top teeth and relaxing the jaw. Spend 15 to 30 seconds warming up the nose. You should notice unlocked nasal pathways and less resistance.

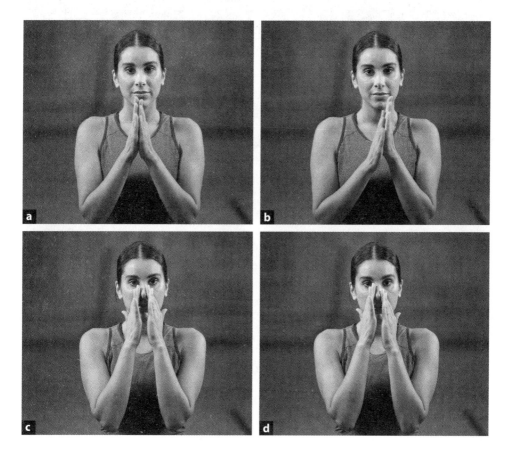

Nostril Pulling

Place your middle finger and index finger at the sides and base of each nostril (see figure *a*). As you inhale, use the pressure of your fingers to lift the nostrils and pull the cheeks (see figure *b*). This manual nasal dilator should allow for a deeper breath. You can either lift for 30 seconds or count breaths. However, it is best to lift the nostrils and take five deep nasal breaths. This allows you to be mindful of each breath and focus on deepening the breathing as well as lengthening the pace of the breath. As the nostrils rise, you should feel an immediate ease in airflow through the nose.

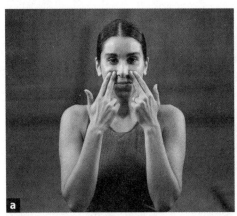
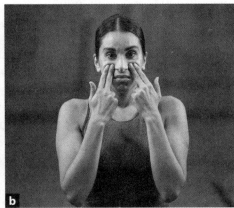

Face Warm-Up

Warming up the face will help you release tension in your face while also stimulating the nervous system and blood flow. As you move through the following exercises, your breathing will become smoother and relaxed as the muscles in the face relax.

Forehead Massage

Place four fingers of each hand near the middle of your forehead (see figure *a*). Imagine you have four lines running across your forehead and press your fingers into them, and pull your fingers across the forehead (see figure *b*). Repeat five times.

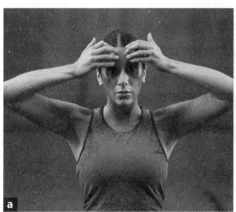 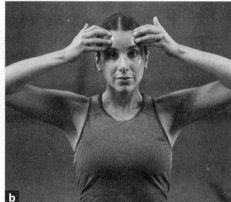

Forehead Rubbing

Rub the palm of your hand back and forth across the forehead until you feel heat on the forehead (see figures *a-b*).

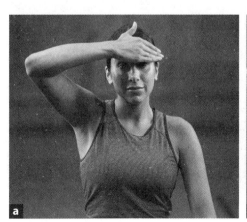 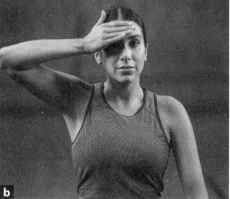

Eye Massage

Use the index finger and middle finger to gently massage the eye area, being careful not to use the fingernails. First, rub below the eyes as you pull the skin toward your ears five times (see figure *a*). Next, rub around the eyes in a complete circle, starting in the middle of the eyebrows and moving around the outer edges of the eyes. Repeat five times (see figures *b-e*).

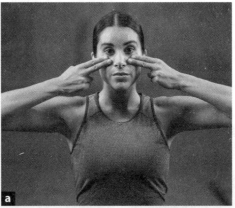

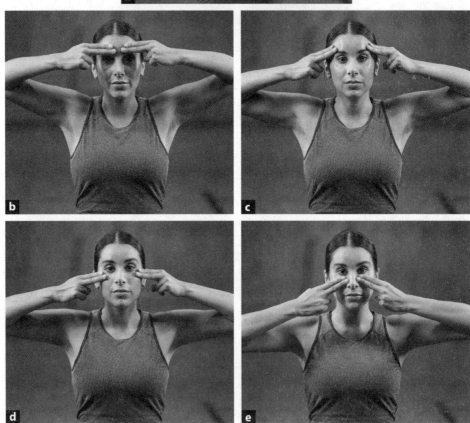

Jaw Massage

With the right thumb, massage the right side of the jaw by applying pressure to the underside of it. Start near the ear and work down the jawline. Move your thumb back and forth for 30 to 90 seconds (see figure *a*). Repeat along the left jaw, using the left thumb. Breathe through the nose calmly and rhythmically. Next, place your thumb under your jaw just below the tongue and push up while pulling the jaw out. Hold this position for 10 seconds while nasal breathing (see figure *b*).

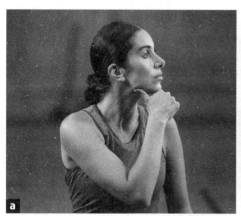 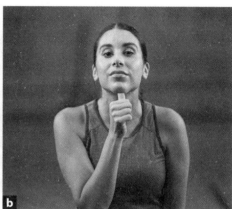

Neck Warm-Up

After warming up the face and nose, it's time to warm up the neck. Rounded shoulders, constant sitting, and forward head posture put a lot of daily stress on the neck. The neck can be overworked during training and competition when the secondary breathing muscles are recruited excessively. Massaging and warming up the neck muscles improves spine posture.

Lymph Node Massage

Use your index and middle finger to rub in a circular motion behind the ears where the jawbone starts (see figure). Rub in clockwise and counterclockwise circles five times in each direction. Breathe through the nose at a calm and rhythmic pace.

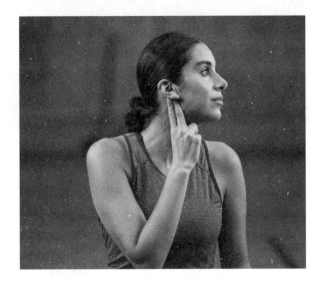

Sternocleidomastoid Massage

The sternocleidomastoid muscle is a large muscle that runs along each side of the neck from the back of the skull to the collarbone. To warm up the sternocleido-mastoid muscle, place the index, middle, and ring fingers at the top of the right side of the neck. With the middle finger as the main point of contact applying the pressure, rub up and down the right side of the neck 10 times (see figure *a*) and then rub side to side 10 times (see figure *b*). Repeat on the left side using the left hand. Breathe calmly through the nose at a rhythmic pace.

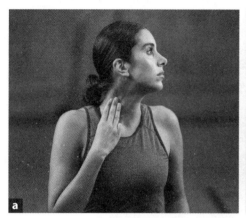 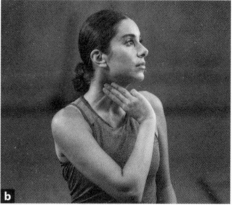

Scalene Massage

The scalenes are three muscles located on each side of the neck and, as accessory breathing muscles, are involved in lifting the first two ribs during a forced inhalation. The scalenes are deeper than the sternocleidomastoid muscle. They attach on each side of the cervical vertabrae and to the first two ribs. To warm up the scalene muscles, massage the left side of the neck with the right hand and the right side of the neck with the left hand. Start at the clavicle and, with the index and middle fingers, massage around the bone (see figure). Move side to side for five to eight seconds, then move up and down for five to eight seconds. Maintain nasal breathing throughout.

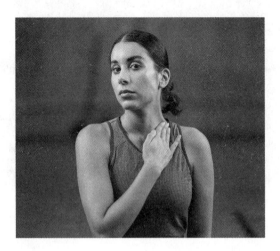

Voice Box Massage

To warm up the voice box area, place the index finger and thumb at the top of the voice box (see figure) to move it side to side gently for three to five repetitions. Repeat at the middle of the voice box and then at the bottom. Breathe rhythmically and slowly through your nose with enough force to make a quiet sound.

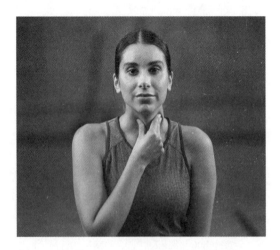

Neck Circle

Pull the shoulders down away from the ears and slowly draw an imaginary circle in the air with your nose. Make the circle as big as you can while maintaining nasal breathing (see figures *a-d*). Make three full circles in one direction and then three full circles in the other.

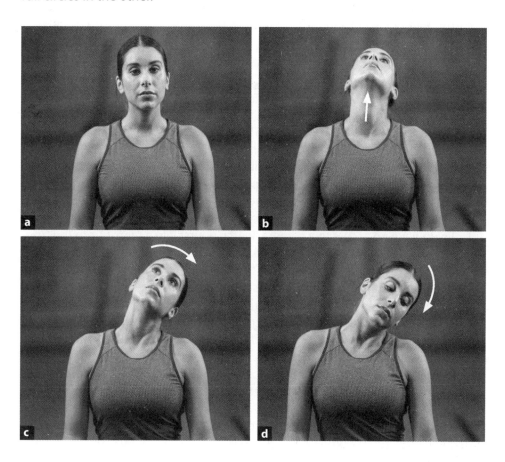

Horizontal Breathing Tests

Proper breathing mechanics are necessary to be able to perform daily activities with ease. The first step in achieving this is to learn horizontal breathing, which expands the rib cage and engages the breathing muscles to support the spine during movement. In addition to protecting the spine, horizontal breathing allows you to maximize the energy gained through the breath.

Rib Cage 360 Test

For optimal exchange of oxygen for carbon dioxide, you must properly use the diaphragm and expand the rib cage during breathing. This supplies the body with the oxygen it needs to perform optimally both mentally and physically.

To learn how to properly use the diaphragm and expand the rib cage, have a coach or trainer record you from the front, side, and back while you are breathing so you can observe yourself from all sides. You can also record yourself if you are able. If you have no access to a camera, watch yourself in a mirror from the front and side while breathing. Men should take their shirt off, and women should wear a sports bra so they can see as much of the body and rib cage as possible. Stand up straight in a relaxed posture and rest your arms at your sides. The goal is to observe your body in a natural position while you're breathing.

Start all observations with nasal breathing and then observe mouth breathing. Take three breaths through the nose, and then take three breaths through the mouth. For each breath, notice what happens in the rib cage and around the center of the body. You should feel the first movement of a nasal breath lower and into the belly. You should feel the first movement of a mouth breath higher and into the upper chest. If you or your coach can't see movement in the body, breathe louder, which will use the muscles more. This exercise helps you recognize the difference between mouth and nose breathing.

Proper mechanics will develop a diaphragm strong enough to create horizontal movement during heavy breathing and mouth breathing in training and competition. You shouldn't see any of the breaths move the upper chest or any part of the body that is above the nipples; the neck and shoulders should not be involved in the breath. The goal is to see lateral movement at the center of the body and minimal upper-body movement. You may notice a difference between the nose and mouth breaths, which is fine. If you are new to breath work, you might breathe shallowly into your shoulders through either your nose or mouth. The exercises in this book teach you how to breathe horizontally into the rib cage rather than vertically into the shoulders. Next, focus your attention on taking slow, deep inhalations and soft, passive exhalations and then observe the movement in your body from the front, side, and back.

Front

Breathe using this cadence: Inhale for three seconds, pause for one second, and then exhale for three seconds. Take three breaths through the nose. As you breathe, you should see the rib cage expand laterally and minimal movement above the nipples (see figure). Repeat by taking three breaths through the mouth.

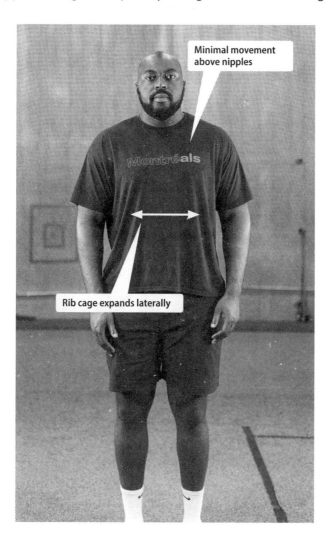

Side

Breathe using this cadence: Inhale for three seconds, pause for one second, and then exhale for three seconds. Take three breaths through the nose. As you breathe, you should see a forward and backward rib movement (see figure). The intercostals should push the ribs out horizontally while you see movement in front of and behind the arms. Repeat by taking three breaths through the mouth.

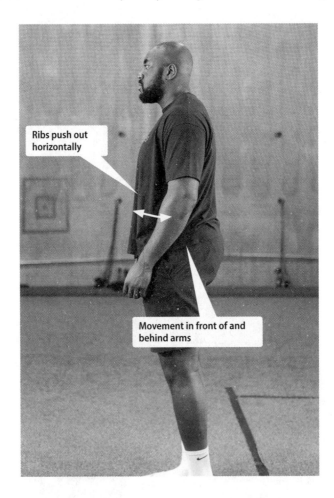

Back

Breathe using this cadence: Inhale for three seconds, pause for one second, and then exhale for three seconds. Take three breaths through the nose. As you breathe, the initial movement should be felt and seen in the middle of the back as the ribs expand (see figure). It can be a struggle to breathe into the back because the bottom ribs are difficult to push out, even when using the diaphragm. Repeat by taking three breaths through the mouth.

Note that this aspect of breathing mechanics may take the longest to master. If you struggle to see movement in the back ribs, practice the back breathing exercises in chapter 7.

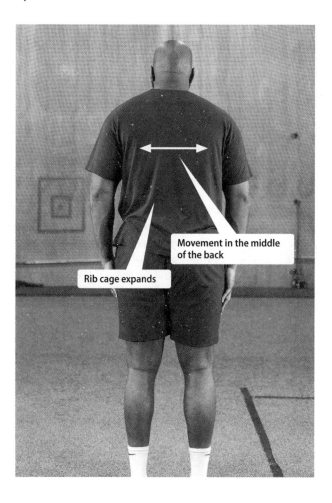

Movement in the middle of the back

Rib cage expands

Using the BIQ Test to Measure Breathing Effectiveness

Dr. Belisa Vranich, a clinical psychologist and author of *Breathing for Warriors*, developed the Breathing IQ (BIQ) Test, which measures the effectiveness of an athlete's breathing. It shows whether an athlete is using their main breathing muscles and whether they are using them correctly. The BIQ score helps an athlete see the location of movement (LOM) and the range of motion (ROM) of the diaphragm.

The first part of the test determines the LOM, or style in which someone is breathing: vertical, horizontal, or hybrid (both). The person being tested takes normal breaths while a coach or trainer observes them or while watching themselves in a mirror. It should be easy to determine a person's breathing style by seeing how their body moves when they take a breath. Dr. Vranich has found that 9 out of 10 adults breathe vertically into their neck and shoulders. A horizontal movement should look like the person is able to breathe 360 degrees around the bottom of the rib cage and a hybrid breather would be a mix between a vertical and horizontal breather.

Once the location of movement has been established, the test measures the range of motion of the diaphragm. To measure this, find the bottom of the rib cage and place a tape measure around the body at the bottom of the rib cage. Measure the circumference of the rib cage after a full inhalation and again after a full exhalation. Use this formula to find the ROM of the diaphragm:

inhalation measurement − (exhalation measurement ÷ exhalation measurement) × 10 = _____ %

The ideal result is a horizontal breather with a score of 80 percent or higher on their ROM test. In her book, Dr. Vranich cites research on breathing showing that by age 29, thoracic flexibility and lung volume have peaked. This means that after the age of 30, unless a breathing element is part of a training program, the amount of oxygen going into and out of the body will decrease (Sharma and Goodwin 2006).

According to Dr. Vranich, "The best way to have strong lungs is to strengthen the muscles that make them fill and empty—the 10 pounds [4.5 kilograms] of inhale and exhale muscles that include the diaphragm, intercostals, and core/ab muscles. Realize that your lungs don't power themselves; you need to do breathing exercises to keep them healthy." The Breathing IQ Test is discussed fully in *Breathing for Warriors*, and a three-minute assessment to measure LOM and ROM of the diaphragm is available at www.thebreathingiq.com.

Lung Volume and Lung Capacity Measurements

The lung volume and lung capacity measurements covered in this section will help you determine the health of your lungs and quality of your daily breathing. This information can help you learn how to handle stress in the body. These measurements are expressed in milliliters (mL). For each type of volume or capacity, a range of values is listed. The higher numbers indicate the average for men, and the lower numbers indicate the average for women. See figure 5.1 for average lung volume and capacity measurements.

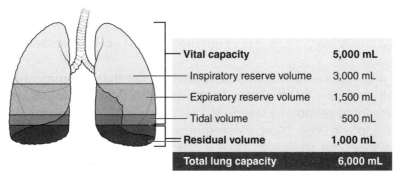

Vital capacity	**5,000 mL**
Inspiratory reserve volume	3,000 mL
Expiratory reserve volume	1,500 mL
Tidal volume	500 mL
Residual volume	**1,000 mL**
Total lung capacity	**6,000 mL**

FIGURE 5.1   Lung volume and capacity measurements.

Lung Volume Measurements

These are the four important lung volume measurements: tidal volume, inspiratory reserve volume, expiratory reserve volume, and residual volume. These measurements reflect lung function and health and can be used to determine whether the lungs are providing peak gas exchange.

Lung volume is measured with a spirometer. A spirometer is a device used by patients after surgery and by people with lung conditions such as COPD and asthma, but it is also useful to athletes. It is the most common device for measuring pulmonary function and breathing capacity, and it helps people practice deep breathing while maximizing the exchange of gases. Lung volumes indicate how well the thoracic cage, respiratory muscles, and lungs are working together to move air in and out. The stronger the breathing muscles, the greater the lung capacity, which leads to higher endurance, mental clarity, and better overall well-being.

Take a look at swimming, for example, the sport that is considered to have the most profound effect on the lungs. A study in 2016 followed swimmers who were using spirometry testing to track the progress of their lung capacity (Lazovic-Popovic et al. 2016). The testing showed that swimmers had higher lung capacity than athletes in other sports and higher than people who lived sedentary lives. The study showcased the use of a spirometer to measure and track progress of the lungs during physical activity and training. Typically, adult men have slightly larger lung volumes than women, and taller people have larger lung volumes than shorter people. The values provided in the drills are averages and should be used simply as a guide. Your age, body type, and lifestyle habits will also come into play.

When using a spirometer, you will perform a series of breaths into a tube. A gauge on the spirometer will display how much air you inhale and exhale. The device should also show how quickly you are able to fill and empty your lungs. Some portable spirometry devices function on their own, while others are paired with a smartphone app. Either one provides a reliable evaluation of the respiratory system.

The results you get from spirometry indicate the strength of your lungs. And as you've learned, your lungs are operated by numerous breathing muscles. Just as it's important to strengthen the muscles used for locomotion and lifting, it is also important to strengthen the breathing muscles.

These are reasons to use a spirometry device:

- Track progress and growth
- Track overall health and lung capacity
- Track endurance levels
- Strengthen the respiratory system

Tidal Volume (TV) Measurement

Tidal volume is the amount of air that you move in and out of your lungs while breathing normally and at rest. To measure the TV, place your mouth over a mouthpiece attached to a spirometer and breathe normally. The average amount of tidal volume a normal human brings in with each inhalation is 300 to 500 mL. Most athletes should be close to this number. The measurement should always be around the average range and show consistency in volume while at rest.

When you are training or competing, the tidal volume and depth of breathing increase. The rate of breathing increases, and this has the effect of taking more oxygen into the body and removing more carbon dioxide. Poor tidal volume limits oxygen consumption in the body and physical compensation in athletic movements. This is caused by overbreathing or poor breathing mechanics. Breathing practices, a strong diaphragm, and physical fitness help maintain your normal tidal volume longer (Hallett, Fadi, and Ashurst 2022).

Inspiratory Reserve Volume (IRV) Measurement

Inspiratory reserve volume is the total amount of air you can inhale above tidal volume. In other words, after a normal breath with a normal tidal volume, you would take a full inhalation and reach peak inhalation. The typical volume for a young adult is 1,900 to 3,000 mL. Your inability to reach full capacity with the inhalation indicates an obstruction or restriction in the airways. While measuring at rest, if you are able to reach full capacity, you should be able to reach into reserves when tidal volume increases.

Expiratory Reserve Volume (ERV) Measurement

Expiratory reserve volume is the total amount of air you can exhale following a forceful exhalation. This is similar to the IRV measurement, but you are forcing out as much air as possible. This forced exhalation follows normal breathing. The typical volume for a young adult is 700 to 1,100 mL. This volume is important because when you run out of air, you can tap into these reserve volumes when tidal volume has increased. Obstructions or restrictions in the airway disrupt your ability to reach these volumes.

Residual Volume (RV) Measurement

Residual volume is the air left in your lungs after exhaling. This air helps keep the lungs from collapsing. It is also important because it prevents large fluctuations in respiratory gases by keeping the exchange of gases continuous even after exhalation. Residual volume is measured after a maximal exhalation. The typical volume for a young adult is about 1,000 mL.

Lung Capacity Measurements

The capacity and health of the lungs directly affects the health of an athlete's cardiorespiratory function, and when you have a healthy and strong cardiorespiratory system, you are able to perform and exercise more efficiently. The larger your lung capacity, the better you are able to get oxygen into the bloodstream and into the working muscles where it is needed for processing energy. The tests in these sections help you understand the capacity and functionality of the lungs. These are the four lung capacity tests: total lung capacity (TLC), vital capacity (VC), inspiratory capacity (IC), and the functional residual capacity (FRC).

Conditions such as COPD, asthma, bronchitis, obesity, and emphysema are the main causes of poor lung capacity. However, weak breathing muscles, poor posture, and overbreathing affect lung capacity and endurance.

Total Lung Capacity (TLC)

Total lung capacity is the measurement of all four lung volumes: tidal volume, inspiratory reserve volume, expiratory reserve volume, residual volume. TLC is important because it is an indicator of general health. A 29-year study showed that a person's lung capacity directly affected their life expectancy (Schünemann et al. 2000). The average TLC range is 4,200 to 6,000 mL. TLC is the sum of the four lung volume measurements:

$$TLC = TV + IRV + ERV + RV$$

Vital Capacity (VC)

Vital capacity (VC) is the total amount of air you can expel following the deepest possible inhalation. This is the maximum amount of air breathed in, followed by the maximum amount of air breathed out. Many factors affect your VC:

- *Height and weight*—Body size affects how much air we can bring in and let out.
- *Sex*—Men have a higher vital capacity than women because their lungs are bigger than women's. Some studies show a 10 to 12 percent difference in lung size, while others show a 25 percent difference. Men's lungs hold about 6 liters of air, while the average woman's lungs hold 4.2 to 4.5 liters (Bellemare, Jeanneret, and Couture 2003).
- *Size of rib cage*—Some people naturally have a wider rib cage, and a larger rib cage allows them to take in more air.
- *Posture*—Poor posture negatively affects vital capacity by limiting the range of motion of the diaphragm and disrupting healthy breathing patterns.
- *Age*—Athletes under the age of 25 have the highest vital capacity.
- *Fitness level*—Higher fitness levels increase vital capacity.

Athletes typically have a higher vital capacity simply because of the amount of physical activity they engage in, and physical activity increases a person's depth of breathing. A higher vital capacity indicates that an athlete has stronger and bigger lungs that can readily expand and take in more air, increasing the uptake of oxygen. The good news is that vital lung capacity can be trained and improved through exercises that make the lungs stronger, such as pursed-lip breathing, deep belly breathing, and interval and resistance training. This makes oxygen more readily available to the brain, heart, and muscles, allowing athletes to perform longer without losing their breath.

The average VC is 3,500 to 5,000 mL and is typically three times the tidal volume (TV). VC is the sum of the tidal volume, inspiratory reserve volume, and expiratory reserve volume:

$$VC = TV + IRV + ERV$$

You can also measure vital capacity using a balloon (use a latex-free balloon if you're allergic to latex). First, stretch the balloon to make it easier to inflate. Next, sit in a chair or on the floor with good posture and take a maximum inhalation followed by a maximum exhalation into the balloon. Force as much air into the balloon as you can in one breath. The volume of air in the balloon is your vital capacity. While pinching the neck of the balloon to keep air from escaping, measure and track the circumference of the balloon by using a marker to draw a line where the balloon begins to expand from the neck. The goal is to over time increase the size of the same balloon with one breath.

Inspiratory Capacity (IC)

Inspiratory capacity is the maximum volume of air you can inhale following a normal, quiet expiration. Weak inspiratory muscles limit lung expansion during inhalation. Fatigue can cause you to hyperventilate or use accessory muscles to inhale. A higher IC allows you to withstand stress and fatigue longer. The average IC is 2,100 to 3,000 mL. IC is the sum of inspiratory reserve volume and tidal volume:

$$IC = IRV + TV$$

Functional Residual Capacity (FRC)

Functional residual capacity should not be confused with residual volume. Functional residual capacity is the volume of air remaining in the lungs after expiration of a normal and passive breath. The functional residual capacity is the residual volume plus the expiratory reserve volume. Without FRC, the gas exchange between oxygen and carbon dioxide would vary wildly and disrupt the diffusion in the lungs. The average FRC is 1,800 to 2,500 mL. FRC is the sum of RV and ERV:

$$FRC = RV + ERV$$

Physiological Stress Tests

The tests in this section will help you create a deeper understanding of how you're handling stress. Mismanaging stress can lead to cognitive fatigue, brain fog, mood swings, anxiety, and lack of energy. These symptoms affect the response to stimulus, which then disrupts the flow state of performance during training and competition.

Markers that indicate an athlete's physiological state are resting heart rate, respiration rate, heart rate variability, and $\dot{V}O_2$max. Some of these can be measured manually, while others require the use of technology. Resting heart rate and heart rate variability (HRV) tests aren't breathing tests; however, they are useful in gauging how an athlete's cardiorespiratory system is reacting to stress. For example, a resting heart rate that is higher than normal can indicate that an athlete has not fully recovered from training or competition. The HRV score, while factoring in heart rate, actually measures how well the autonomic nervous system is helping the body recover from stress. While these two heart rate measurements are important, this section will focus primarily on tracking the exhalation length and breath-holding scores.

Resting Heart Rate

Resting heart rate (RHR) is the measurement of how many times your heart beats per minute when you are at rest. Your RHR is a reliable indicator of your state of recovery. Heart rate devices and trackers are available, but you can also measure RHR by taking a few seconds to breathe calmy through the nose, then lightly press two fingers to the neck to feel your pulse at the carotid artery. Count the number of beats in 15 seconds and multiply that by four. The result is your resting heart rate.

Measure your RHR each morning within the first hour of being awake and record it. Focus on measuring during the same conditions each morning. For example, always before getting out of bed. Study your data for a month. You may find that your resting heart rate is higher after strenuous competition or training than it is after days when you weren't overly stressed. Other factors that can affect RHR are quality of sleep, diet, and changing time zones and climate while traveling. Emotional and mental stress can also affect RHR.

After consistently tracking your RHR for two or more weeks that include a typical number of hard and easy training days, find your average RHR (sum of daily heart rate divided by number of days). Use your RHR to learn how you're handling the stress of training and competition. An RHR that is slightly below your average means you're recovering well and are ready for additional stress. If the RHR is high, especially unusually high, you need to focus on recovery instead of training.

Respiration Rate

The resting respiratory rate is a vital sign often affected by stressors such as emotional tension, cognitive load, heat, cold, physical stress, and fatigue. It is crucial in gauging how you are handling stress. Ideally, the respiratory rate should be low and consistent. A normal resting respiratory rate for an average adult is 12 to 20 breaths per minute. Breathing faster than 24 breaths per minute can lead to serious health issues, although the health issue may be less serious if the rate of respiration increases because of psychological factors such as a panic attack.

Respiratory rate is measured at rest and counts the number of breaths taken per minute. While using a stopwatch or clock to keep track of time, breathe normally and count a full inhalation and exhalation as one breath. Breathe through the nose and focus on keeping the breathing pace natural. Several wearable devices measure respiration rate.

Heart Rate Variability (HRV)

Heart rate variability is the variation in the time between heart beats. During an ideal recovery scenario, this interval fluctuates slightly. Many coaches and trainers use HRV scores to determine when an athlete is recovered. A high HRV score indicates a lack of stress or fatigue. When you are relaxed and recovered, your HRV is higher. This would mean you have greater variability between heart beats. When the body and mind are recovering from stress or intense exercise, the HRV is lower, which means you have less variability between heart beats. Pushing through a low readiness score can lead to injury and illness. There is no way to measure HRV without equipment. The most accurate way to measure HRV is through an EKG. However, many reliable wearable devices are available.

$\dot{V}O_2$max

$\dot{V}O_2$max is the maximum volume ($\dot{V}$) of oxygen (O_2) the body can process and quantifies the body's capacity to use oxygen when exercising. The higher the $\dot{V}O_2$max, the greater the capacity to do work. $\dot{V}O_2$max has three primary components:

- *Lung capacity and heart volume*—The more oxygen the lungs can take in, the more oxygenated blood the heart can pump. This will create a max $\dot{V}O_2$ score.
- *Capillary delivery*—More oxygenated blood entering the circulatory system transports more oxygen into the muscles. This affects $\dot{V}O_2$max.
- *Muscle efficiency*—The better muscles can extract and use oxygen from blood, the higher the $\dot{V}O_2$max.

Knowing your $\dot{V}O_2$max establishes a fitness baseline from which to track improvement and determine the effectiveness of your training. If your $\dot{V}O_2$max is low, you might struggle through low to moderate aerobic exercise and should review your breathing mechanics and training system. A higher $\dot{V}O_2$max will give you better endurance so you're able to sustain a faster pace during aerobic activity. Many coaches and trainers feel this test is the best way to measure aerobic endurance and cardiovascular fitness. Numerous studies show that higher aerobic fitness is linked to improved quality of life, longer life span, overall better mood and self-esteem, and improved sleep patterns.

The most accurate way to test $\dot{V}O_2$max is in a laboratory in a sports medicine facility or medical facility. Athletes breathe into an oxygen mask and walk on a treadmill at a certain pace for a certain time. $\dot{V}O_2$max can also be measured on wearable tracking devices. Another option is to pair an online or manual calculator with an aerobic test: 1-mile (1.6 km) walk, three-minute step test, 1.5-mile (2.4 km) run, or 2,000-meter rowing. The calculation to determine $\dot{V}O_2$max uses age, gender, weight, the amount of time it takes to complete the test, and pulse rate during the test. Instructions for the tests can be found online.

You can improve your $\dot{V}O_2$max through breathing exercises and improve your cardiorespiratory system without doing traditional cardio exercises. Start by establishing horizontal breathing and then implement breath-holding exercises and engage in low to moderate exercise while breathing through the nose only (three to five times a week).

Exhale Test

The exhale test measures the length of an exhalation. The longer the exhalation, the greater the tolerance of carbon dioxide, the stress messenger of the body. Athletes with longer exhalation times are better recovered and in a better readiness state. You can take this measurement any time you experience mental and physical stress to help you determine your readiness state.

To complete the test, sit with a stopwatch and breathe slowly through the nose for at least one minute to bring the body to a state of calmness. Once you feel you are calm and you are breathing at a steady rhythm, begin the test. Take three focused breaths with inhalations and exhalations longer than normal. These three breaths are not meant to reach maximum inhalation and exhalation, but are bigger than normal breaths. After the third exhalation, take a maximum inhalation. At the top of the inhalation, pause briefly. Following the pause, start the watch at the beginning of the exhalation and measure the full length of a smooth, uninterrupted exhalation. Exhale through the nose as slowly as possible. This should feel like the air is slowly leaking out through the nose. Do not rush or push the air out. Stop the watch when you have released all the air.

You should be able to exhale for at least 20 seconds. Less than 20 seconds indicates a low tolerance to carbon dioxide, which can result in overbreathing and anxiety. An exhalation shorter than 20 seconds could also indicate sickness or injury. Shorter exhalation scores indicate an inability to mechanically breathe well and a low tolerance to carbon dioxide. With training, you should be able to extend an exhalation by 30 to 50 seconds. As you increase your tolerance to carbon dioxide, you should be able to exhale for 60 to 80 seconds or even longer. Test this every two weeks to track how you are adapting to training and competitive atmospheres.

Breath-Hold Tests

These final two tests, which measure how long you can hold your breath, provide direct feedback on how you handle stress and your capacity to self-regulate. Holding the breath can induce a sense of panic, so it is important to see how well you handle this stress from a physiological and psychological standpoint. As the respiratory centers become less sensitive to breath holding over time, you will find it easier to withstand the stress buildup. This is why it is important to consistently practice and improve your breath-holding times (later chapters will showcase many breath-holding exercises).

When you hold your breath, the volume of oxygen decreases and the volume of carbon dioxide increases. Although you can feel this while holding your breath, some people benefit from watching this happen on the display of a pulse oximeter. They follow their SpO_2 (peripheral capillary). A benefit to dropping the SpO_2 below 90 percent (a normal reading is typically 95 to 100 percent) is that it simulates the experience of being at high altitude and naturally creates more red bloods cells. A pulse oximeter is not necessary for the tests in this chapter, but it may be easier to make consistent progress by using one during your breath-holding exercises. You can also use it to make sure you're not dropping too low (e.g., 60 or 70 percent).

During the two tests in this section, you may not be able to hold your breath long enough to register a drop in saturation levels, especially if you're new to breath holding. Most people don't see oxygen saturation drop until two to three minutes of retention, and even then it depends on a variety of individual factors. So you may want to save the use of the pulse oximeter for exercises such as max breath holds or any breath hold that follows a hyperventilation breathing technique. The device is also helpful in tracking oxygen levels and comparing the drop with how you feel and how long it takes for your oxygen levels to change.

Exhale Breath-Hold Test

This test measures your tolerance to carbon dioxide buildup after an exhalation hold. It is based on a breath-holding assessment called the BOLT (body oxygen level test) developed by Patrick McKeown, an author, researcher, and breathing coach (who we highlighted in chapter 3). This test focuses on a controlled nasal inhalation following an exhalation hold. If you will perform high-altitude or breath-hold training, you should be able to hold your breath for longer than 20 seconds on this test.

To perform this test, breathe normally through the nose for one minute. Normal breathing is silent nasal breathing with minimal movement in the body. Following the minute of focused normal breathing, exhale naturally and hold your breath by pinching the nose, closing the mouth, and closing the eyes. Start the watch and hold your breath until you feel a strong sense of stress and the need to breathe.

At this point, stop the watch. The first inhalation must be through the nose as a recovery breath. If the first inhalation after the hold is through the mouth, restart because this means you have held your breath too long. The goal is to maintain normal breathing throughout the test and a measured hold following exhalation. This will indicate when you reach breathlessness. As you are able to hold your breath longer in this test, you will experience breathlessness less often.

Inhale Breath-Hold Test

This test measures the length of your breath hold on an inhalation. It is similar to the previous test, except it measures the length of your breath hold on an inhalation instead of an exhalation. The hold is less stressful because the lungs are more full after an inhalation. The inhale-hold test is not as mentally difficult, and you may be able to hold your breath longer.

Similar to the exhale test, breathe entirely through the nose for one minute to calm the nervous system. Once you are settled and breathing normally for a minute and find your natural rhythm, take a normal inhalation and hold the breath by pinching the nose, closing the mouth, and closing the eyes. Start the watch and hold your breath until you feel a strong sense of stress and the need to breathe. The first exhalation must be let out through the nose as a recovery breath. If the first exhalation after the hold is through the mouth, restart because you have held your breath too long. The goal is to maintain normal breathing during the test and a measured hold following inhalation.

Athletes can typically hold their breath from 30 seconds to two minutes. If you can hold your breath for over a minute but find it difficult to on a specific day, you are probably stressed, fatigued, or sick. Use this test to keep tabs on your health, recovery, and readiness state.

My hope is that you now have a deeper understanding of what happens in your body and mind with each breath. Learning how you should breathe and being able to see proper body movement in yourself and others are crucial. Beyond the mechanics of breathing, knowing how the lung volume and capacity function for each breath allows you to maximize the exchange of gases. Without proper exchange of oxygen and carbon dioxide, your endurance and overall well-being are minimized. If you find value in using technology, you can choose from a variety of devices to help you monitor cardiorespiratory function to improve performance. When using manual measuring techniques and tests, pay attention to how you feel and how you're responding to a particular workload during the tests and during training and competition. If your resting heart rate is high, your respiratory rate is high, or you're having trouble extending an exhalation or holding your breath, chances are you are not sufficiently adapting to stress. Your goal as an athlete is to optimize the space between stimulus and response by providing opportunity for flow to control performance. For this to happen, you must be able to manage and conquer your stress through optimal adaptation. Slow and controlled breathing outside of training and competitive environments along with flexibility and freedom in the mind to handle breath holding indicate that you are in a positive physiological and psychological state. As you move into breathing practices and the exercises in this book, keep in mind that you are the highest form of technology when it comes to knowing yourself.

6

Oxygenation Exercises

By now, you understand what effective breathing mechanics are and how consistency in positive breathing habits improves the nervous system and calms the mind. You have also learned the value of breathing more slowly and how breathing through the nose keeps the body and mind oxygenated, which are keys for optimal performance. The exercises in this chapter will help you increase energy levels and sustain them over the course of your training year.

Monitoring sensations is important in oxygenation breath practices. Much of the oxygenation training through breath work includes breath holds, which means these exercises include a psychological component. Breath holding causes a feeling of suffocation, which can trigger a sense of anxiety and panic. Please note that if these exercises create extremely high levels of anxiety or stress, then this type of breath training will not work. Breath work should not negatively affect the system. Some exercises will work well for certain people but won't work at all for others. So try exercises until you find those that work for you.

The previous chapter provided inhalation and exhalation breath-holding tests. The initial test results provide a baseline from which to measure progress in increasing the amount of time you can hold your breath, improving how well you tolerate stress, and improving your ability to calm your mind. The breath-holding tests also prepare you for the more involved breath-holding practices in this chapter.

Breathing improvements, whether mechanical or physiological, will most likely occur exponentially as you begin focused breath work. As you improve your exhalation test scores, your breath holds will get longer naturally as you begin breathing properly throughout the day. When you are intentional and curious about breathing you will get better at perceiving when you are breathing too fast, either by recognizing the movements in the body or that you are mouth breathing. You can quickly make adjustments throughout the day that will lead to improvements in performance. The body naturally adapts to healthy breathing by handling higher levels of carbon dioxide buildup, which naturally lowers the respiratory rate and increases endurance. These positive adaptations will further extend an exhalation and breath-holding times during retesting.

Once your diaphragm is moving properly, you've become aware of your daily breathing habits, and you can focus on slow breathing and implementing a few breath exercises, you'll experience new levels of energy and improved recovery. Remember that as you improve, the rate of progress will slow. It's similar to the process of committing to the weight room. Strength at first increases quickly and over time slows. Don't feel discouraged if you go from a 20-second exhalation to a 70-second exhalation in a month and then make less improvement the following month. The exhalation test and amount of time you can hold your breath will hit a peak. However, once your breathing scores have peaked, you have established strong habits and routines, and proper breathing has become a practice of consistency rather than a practice of progress.

Consistency executed over time will produce noticeable results and eventually lead to healthy subconscious behaviors. Use these exercises to build a deeper understanding of yourself and how well you are adapting to stressors in your life both in and outside of performance. From this foundation you will experience better recovery, sustainable energy, and a deeper sense of self both mentally and physically. Breathing is your guide to reaching your athletic performance potential. You may progress quickly, but adaptation is a long-term process that requires consistency.

Reminder: If the breathing exercises cause dizziness, lightheadedness, or the feeling that you might faint, stop immediately and begin slow breathing to calm your system.

Buteyko Breathing Technique

The Buteyko breathing technique (BBT), or Buteyko method, uses breath-retention practice to control the breath so that you breathe more slowly and with more volume. It was established in the 1950s by physiologist Konstantin Buteyko in Russia as a therapeutic treatment to help asthma patients prevent coughing, wheezing, and feeling short of breath. The technique was also established to help people with anxiety to slow their breathing. It is still used as a nonpharmacological intervention for these issues. A 2008 study showed that people with asthma who used this technique reduced their need for inhaled corticosteroid therapy (Cowie et al. 2008). The technique helps people who overbreathe or hyperventilate to establish breath awareness, strengthen nasal breathing, and train the body to breathe more slowly. Some find that this technique can clear nasal passages and clogged nostrils.

As an athlete, you want functional breathing patterns that feel light and effortless to happen unconsciously throughout the day. If you yawn or sigh frequently, this might occur because you feel as though you're not getting enough air and take bigger breaths to compensate and stop the fatigue. The Buteyko method is a great way to balance breathing, eliminate upper-chest breathing, and alleviate yawning and sighing. If you experience asthma or nasal obstruction, the Buteyko method will improve flow through the airways and ease breathing.

This method uses breath retention to slow the off-loading process of excess carbon dioxide. As the breath slows and you begin breath-holding patterns, the body will begin building up carbon dioxide. The ability to handle carbon dioxide buildup benefits performance by keeping you from hyperventilating or over-breathing. When you aren't as reactive to the carbon dioxide buildup that comes from training or overbreathing during the day, you won't experience breathless-ness or fatigue as often. Poor breathing patterns reduce oxygen delivery and narrow the airways, which leads to chronic fatigue. If you are unable to change this, not only will you experience fatigue, yawning, sighing, and exercise-induced asthma but also mental distortion such as anxiety and reacting emotionally. Peak performance cannot be achieved when you are experiencing these symptoms.

To perform BBT, sit cross-legged on the floor or on a chair with the feet flat on the ground. Elongate your spine, maintain an upright posture, and relax your body. Begin by calming the system so you enter the practice in a parasympathetic state. Spend 5 to 10 minutes slowly breathing through the nose at a pace of 5.5 seconds in and 5.5 seconds out with a natural pause after both the inhalation and the exhalation. Once you are calm, focus your attention on extending the spine slightly on each inhalation and then slowly letting the exhalation out softly as you notice the ribs coming back down and the body deflating. This effortless breathing should feel calm, easy, and silent.

After the body reaches equilibrium, start the practice. This exercise is passive and should be done in sync with your natural breathing patterns. To begin, keep the mouth shut and breathe naturally through the nose. When you're ready, exhale and pinch your nostrils shut with your index finger and thumb. The remaining instructions depend on whether you will participate in light activity or heavy activity on the day you perform this protocol. Light activity would include stretching, walking, or low-resistance biking or jogging, for example. In these activities, you are maintaining a low heart rate and feeling minimal stress. Heavy activity would include high-intensity interval training, sprinting, heavy lifts, or plyometrics, for example. These activities will most likely cause mouth breathing, high heart rate, and feelings of fatigue.

- *On lighter-activity days*, hold your breath until you feel the urge to breathe, which may include an involuntary movement of your dia-phragm. Once you feel the urge to breathe, inhale slowly and through the nose. Then breathe normally for a minimum of 10 seconds and maximum of 30 seconds and repeat 10 times. Perform a light-activity breath-hold-ing practice two or three times a week.

- *On heavy-activity days*, hold your breath until you feel the strongest urge to breathe, which may include an involuntary movement of your diaphragm. Once you feel the strong urge to breathe, inhale through the nose. This inhalation may not be slow and might be more intense because you're holding until you feel a strong need to breathe. Then breathe normally for a minimum of 20 seconds and maximum of 40 seconds and repeat 10 times. The hold on a heavy day should be at least twice as long as you held your breath on a lighter day. Perform a heavy-activity breath-holding practice once a week.

Remember, the first inhalation after the hold must be controlled and through the nose. Using only the nose during this practice makes it difficult to take this exercise too far and lose the intention of the exercise. For example, if you feel like you must take a big mouth breath after an exhalation hold, you held the breath too long and the practice was too stressful. Do not focus on long, stressful breath holds, but instead on a controlled and adaptive practice that uses the same natural rhythm as when you started the exercise.

After the hold, the breaths should be gentle and light through the nose to calm your body and return the breathing rate to its natural flow. If you experience anxiety or discomfort, end the practice and continue to breathe normally. Remind yourself to stay mindful of the breath holds. As time goes on, it will become easier to hold the breath for longer periods. Your level of experience and commitment to the practice will have a major impact on your breath-holding abilities. You must have enough experience to fully comprehend the sensations that come with breath holding so you can maintain control, and you must have established a "why" that will sustain your focus and commitment to the practice.

When you begin BBT training, practice in the morning or before athletic training or competition three times a week for six weeks to create a baseline. Once your BBT practice is consistent for six weeks, implement lighter and heavier days into your training programs intuitively. This means you will choose the practice based on what your body tells you it needs instead of based on your athletic training for that day. A 2008 study found that this protocol was effective in lowering respiration rates in people with asthma (Cowie et al. 2008). Even if you are not experiencing a health issue, shortness of breath, coughing, or wheezing, this technique will build a foundation for breath and an awareness of carbon dioxide buildup in the body. It is also an active way to create a mental space for meditation, energy, and focus. While gaining cognitive benefits, you can also slightly improve your endurance and carbon dioxide tolerance while practicing the Buteyko method and achieve a lower respiration rate.

Static Breath-Hold Training

Static breath holding is practiced without movement. It requires more endurance than the Buteyko method and adds stimulus. After you're comfortable with the Buteyko method, practice the static breath holds presented here before moving on to the breath holds with movement. During static breath holding it is easier to time the length of the holds and become mindful within the experience.

In static breath holding you hold your breath for as long as you can in a controlled fashion with the goal to push deeper into breath holding and improve lung capacity for athletic performance. Static breath holding will help you use more of your lungs while controlling the diaphragm. Using more of your lung capacity will not only improve your fitness levels, but you will also find it easier to control your breathing under pressure. Proof of this can be found in the free-diving community. These divers are able to manage and handle stress because they can use their entire lungs and control their mind under pressure. Dives vary in depth but anywhere from 20 to 60 feet is considered an average free dive. Free divers can and will hold their breath for minutes while being underwater.

The free-diving community and surfing community practice a variety of protocols to strengthen their ability to remain calm and relaxed during apnea, or breath holding. Because of the exceptionally long times that free divers hold their breath, they must train this ability. Although most athletes don't need to train breath holding to this extent, these protocols and the teachings can be implemented by any athlete in any sport. One of the best ways to improve this skill is through dry static breath holds. The term *dry* refers to taking place on land, and *static* means without movement. These practices are beneficial for controlling respiratory frequency, handling high-intensity training, dealing with low levels of oxygen in the body, and keeping calm under pressure. World record holder and free diver Stig Severinsen's lungs can hold 14 liters of air. For context, the average male holds 6 liters of air. He attributes this to the breathing exercises he does to increase the length of time he can hold his breath. A study on free divers showed that they experienced significantly lower levels of stress and anxiety than people who do not free dive (Alkan and Akis 2013). Free diving shows the power of the human body and more specifically the breath. By learning from the free-diving community, you can build the power within yourself.

The static breath-hold protocols here strengthen the inspiratory and expiratory muscles. Think of them as miniworkouts to be used on off days or before a training session. The main goal is to increase the breath-hold times and become more comfortable with the sensations that come with holding your breath. Over time you should feel naturally calmer, both in and out of training and competition. You should feel your endurance rise and your ability to recover improve. Each protocol will feel different, so practice them all at first to experience the different sensations. The protocol that fits you best is the protocol that feels the best. Each protocol will be briefly described along with its purpose.

For most healthy athletes, dry static breath holding is safe when practiced in a safe environment. A safe environment is an open space with a soft surface such as a mat, grass, or sand. If you faint or become unconscious and fall, the last thing you want is an injury because of the environment. It is important, however, to be aware that breath holding can lead to increased blood pressure, increased risk of brain damage, loss of coordination, lower heart rate, and increased blood sugar levels (Andersson, Linér, and Jönsson 2009). This section also provides underwater static breath-holding practices for experienced athletes who have mastered the dry static breath-hold practices. Because underwater breath holding presents the risk of losing consciousness underwater and drowning, these practices should be supervised and performed in a shallow pool, 100-gallon (378 liter) tub, bucket of water, or place you can easily stand up or simply lift your face out of the water.

Static Breath-Holding Tips

Consistent breath holding is a skill and a great tool when you want to raise your game and steady your mind. Beyond the performance improvement, it can also offer spiritual benefits. Here are a few things to consider while performing breath-holding protocols:

- *Use whichever is most appropriate during static breath holding: the nose or the mouth.* While nasal breathing is the main resource for breathing, it may be better to use the mouth when you begin breath holding because you are able to bring more air in and move more air out. As your hold times increase or breath holding causes more stress, you can use the mouth to recover.
- *Extend your exhalations so they are longer than the inhalations.* This will decrease the heart rate, calm the mind and body, and consume less oxygen, which means you will be able to hold your breath longer.
- *Pause after each inhalation and exhalation.* The pause must be passive, without stress within the pause and no strain in the diaphragm or intercostal muscles. Pauses decrease the breathing and heart rates.
- *Remain as relaxed as possible.* Relaxation means control when it comes to breath holding. You should feel calm and prepared for each breath hold. Relaxed breathing keeps you calm during the hold.
- *Completely exhale before the inhalation and hold.* Pull the abdominal muscles in as much as possible to push as much air out as you can.

Static Breath-Hold Warm-Up

Warm up before performing the static breath-hold protocols. This warm-up helps you get in touch with your breathing while maintaining a neutral nervous system and homeostasis. To warm up, perform cadenced breathing for five minutes as follows:

- Inhale through the nose for 5.5 seconds.
- Exhale through the nose for 5.5 seconds.
- Take a natural pause after each inhalation and exhalation.
- Repeat for 5 minutes.

Static Breath Holds for High Levels of Carbon Dioxide

Three breath-hold protocols can help the body become accustomed to high levels of carbon dioxide. Each time a protocol decreases the duration of rest, the exercise is meant to build the levels of carbon dioxide. Breath holding can be used on off days as a recovery tool or used before training to prepare the body for stress and challenge the mind. The protocols last 10 to 30 minutes and can be used two to four times a week. Use the easy to moderate protocol on training days and the advanced protocol on off days. These protocols pair well with a sauna and cold exposure (covered in chapter 9). In these three protocols, the breath is held on an inhalation.

Protocol 1: Customized

In this individualized protocol, the length of the hold is based on the result of your inhale breath-hold test in chapter 5. Each hold is 50 percent of your inhale breath-hold time. This creates minimal stress on the mind and body while decreasing the rest period as you move through the protocol. This protocol should take 10 to 15 minutes. Use the full protocol on off days, and on training days, you can use just the first step with 1 minute rest.

Sit on a chair with your feet flat on the ground or sit crossed-legged on the floor. If either of these positions is uncomfortable, you can lie on your back with your knees bent and feet on the floor. Keep a neutral spine in either position. Before holding your breath, exhale all the air before taking a deep horizontal inhalation.

1. 50 percent inhale hold five times, with 1-minute rest between each hold
2. 50 percent inhale hold with 45-second rest
3. 50 percent inhale hold with 30-second rest
4. 50 percent inhale hold with 15-second rest

Protocol 2: Easy to Moderate

Because this protocol is easy to moderate, most people should be able to perform it, regardless of experience level, and it is a good way to start a breath-holding practice. It should not tax the body or mind and can simulate a workout. The holds in this protocol last 40 seconds until the final hold, which lasts at least a minute. The resting time is the only change in this protocol. After each set, you have less time to recover and control your breathing. This protocol will take roughly 10 minutes and can be performed on off days or twice a week before a training session.

Sit on a chair with your feet flat on the ground or sit crossed-legged on the floor. If either of these positions is uncomfortable, lie on your back with your knees bent and feet on the floor. Keep a neutral spine in either position. Before holding your breath, exhale all the air before taking a deep horizontal inhalation.

1. 90 seconds of breathing in and out; inhale and hold for 40 seconds.
2. 60 seconds of breathing in and out; inhale and hold for 40 seconds.
3. 45 seconds of breathing in and out; inhale and hold for 40 seconds.
4. 30 seconds of breathing in and out; inhale and hold for 40 seconds.
5. 15 seconds of breathing in and out; inhale and hold for 40 seconds.
6. Three breaths in and out; inhale and hold for 40 seconds.
7. One breath in and out; inhale and hold for 40 seconds.
8. One breath in and out; inhale and hold for 60 seconds or more.

Protocol 3: Advanced

Before performing this protocol, you should be able to hold your breath for at least 90 seconds. The goal is to hold the breath for 90 seconds and then adequately recover between sets as the resting time decreases. This protocol takes 20 to 25 minutes to complete and consists of eight cycles. Use this protocol only on off days and try to decrease the resting point over time. An appropriate goal is to keep the breath hold at 90 seconds while finishing with one to three breaths in a recovery set.

Sit on a chair with your feet flat on the ground or sit crossed-legged on the floor. If either of these positions is uncomfortable, lie on your back with your knees bent and feet on the floor. Keep a neutral spine in either position. Before holding your breath, exhale all the air before taking a deep horizontal inhalation.

1. Hold breath for 90 seconds.
2. Rest 2 minutes; inhale and hold for 90 seconds.
3. Rest 1:45 minutes; inhale and hold for 90 seconds.
4. Rest 90 seconds; inhale and hold for 90 seconds.
5. Rest 75 seconds; inhale and hold for 90 seconds.
6. Rest 60 seconds; inhale and hold for 90 seconds.
7. Rest 45 seconds; inhale and hold for 90 seconds.
8. Rest 30 seconds; inhale and hold for 90 seconds.

Static Breath Holds for Low Levels of Oxygen

This is a moderate to difficult protocol that accustoms the body to low levels of oxygen by lengthening the duration of the breath holds between resting periods. In this protocol, hold the breath on an inhalation. Use this protocol on an off day as a form of training. It will take about 30 minutes to complete.

Sit on a chair with your feet flat on the ground or sit crossed-legged on the floor. If either of these positions is uncomfortable, lie on your back with your knees bent and feet on the floor. Keep a neutral spine in either position. Before holding your breath, exhale all the air before taking a deep horizontal inhalation.

1. Hold breath for 30 seconds.
2. Rest 2 minutes; inhale and hold for 45 seconds.
3. Rest 2 minutes; inhale and hold for 1 minute.
4. Rest 2 minutes; inhale and hold for 1 minute and 15 seconds.
5. Rest 2 minutes; inhale and hold for 1 minute and 30 seconds.
6. Rest 2 minutes; inhale and hold for 1 minute and 45 seconds.
7. Rest 2 minutes; inhale and hold for 2 minutes.
8. Rest 2 minutes; inhale and hold for 2 minutes and 15 seconds.
9. Rest 2 minutes; inhale and hold for 2 minutes and 30 seconds.

Underwater Static Breath Holds

During the underwater protocols, you will submerge your head. Remember, this can be dangerous and should be practiced in a safe environment with supervision. Using the water to practice breath holding promotes a meditative experience. The water decreases sensory stimulation and helps you relax deeper into the breath holding. It can be a wonderful experience while improving breath-holding ability.

Wear goggles that cover your eyes and nose so you don't have to worry about water getting into your eyes and having to plug your nose. Breathe through the mouth during these protocols and hold the breath on an inhalation. Perform these underwater protocols on off days as a miniworkout and recovery session or perform them once or twice a week before a training session.

Protocol 1: Underwater Static Breath-Hold for High Levels of Carbon Dioxide

In this protocol the rest times decrease, which will help you become accustomed to carbon dioxide buildup. This protocol takes about 10 minutes to complete.

While holding your breath underwater, you will perform a dead man's float. Lie facedown in the water with your arms out to the sides or forward and legs extended back. If you can't make the hold times, come up for air and recover. And do not try the next level if you have trouble completing any of the holds. Perform this protocol using holding times you are comfortable with until you can increase the time.

1. 90 seconds of breathing in and out; inhale and hold for 40 seconds.
2. 60 seconds of breathing in and out; inhale and hold for 40 seconds.
3. 45 seconds of breathing in and out; inhale and hold for 40 seconds.
4. 30 seconds of breathing in and out; inhale and hold for 40 seconds.
5. 15 seconds of breathing in and out; inhale and hold for 40 seconds.
6. Three breaths in and out; inhale and hold for 40 seconds.
7. One breath in and out; inhale and hold for 40 seconds.
8. One breath in and out; inhale and hold for 60 seconds or more.

Protocol 2: Underwater Static Breath Hold for Low Levels of Oxygen

In this protocol, the rest time stays the same while the holds get longer. This will cause stress as you experience low oxygen levels while underwater. Perform this practice on off days as a miniworkout and recovery session, or perform it once a week before a training session. Because the breath holds in this protocol are longer than those in protocol 1, don't attempt this one until you have completed protocol 1 and have experience holding your breath underwater. This will take about 30 minutes to complete.

While holding your breath underwater, you will perform a dead man's float. Lie facedown in the water with your arms out to the sides or forward and legs extended back. If you can't make the hold times, come up for air and recover.

And do not try the next level if you have trouble completing any of the holds. Perform this protocol using holding times you are comfortable with until you can increase the time.

1. Hold breath for 30 seconds.
2. Rest 2 minutes; inhale and hold for 45 seconds.
3. Rest 2 minutes; inhale and hold for 1 minute.
4. Rest 2 minutes; then inhale and hold for 1 minute and 15 seconds.
5. Rest 2 minutes; then inhale and hold for 1 minute and 30 seconds.
6. Rest 2 minutes; then inhale and hold for 1 minute and 30 seconds.
7. Rest 2 minutes; then inhale and hold for 1 minute and 45 seconds.
8. Rest 2 minutes; then inhale and hold for 1 minute and 45 seconds.

Hypoxic Breath Training

The protocols in this section explore hypoxic breath training, which simulates breathing at high altitude, where the oxygen levels are much lower. Of course, the simplest and easiest way to practice these is to actually be at high altitude, but not all athletes have access to the top of a mountain.

The concept of hypoxic breathing is simple. High-altitude environments have less oxygen, and when an athlete lives or trains at high altitude, they acquire more red blood cells, which allows them to carry more oxygen in the blood. This happens because being at high altitude triggers hormonal responses that enhance the way oxygen is delivered to the body. These responses strengthen blood vessels and allow for more blood flow, which improve the heart functionality to enhance muscular performance and in general greater well-being. Sea level air is 20.9 to 21 percent oxygen, while air at 8,000 feet (2,438 meters) is only 15.5 percent oxygen. The drop in oxygen triggers the kidneys to produce erythropoietin (EPO), which stimulates red blood cells in the bone marrow to oxygenate the body. Additionally, the partial pressure of oxygen in the air is less. This means there is less oxygen in the blood for your muscles, heart, and lungs to use. This type of training over time increases endurance at sea level.

The following protocols use breath holds on the exhalation, causing immediate stress because of carbon dioxide and lactic acid buildup in the body. These protocols also use movement to increase the stress. The movement causes the carbon dioxide to build up more quickly, making breath holding more difficult and creating a higher stress stimulus. To manage the stress, ensure that you reach full recovery between sets.

Integrate hypoxic breath-holding training into your program two to four times a week. If you're doing an endurance day, pick an endurance exercise. If you're doing an agility day, pick an agility exercise. If you're doing a strength day, pick a strength exercise. The objective is to perform one clean set of 6 to 10 reps while holding your breath. These breathing exercises should prepare you for a great training session afterward. Train consistently for four to six weeks and then take two weeks off before resuming hypoxic breath-hold training. Track your progress by noting how long you hold your breath or how far you move. You should notice improvement around weeks four to six.

Note that the carbon dioxide buildup in the body during exhalation breath holding can make you feel claustrophobic or like your heart is racing, or it can cause anxiety. You may also feel like your vision is narrowing at the peak of a breath hold. It is normal to feel uncomfortable, but if you feel unsafe, decrease the distance of the movement, the number of reps, or the time for the hold. Exhale naturally rather than forcing as much air from the lungs as you can. Performing the movement with some air in the lungs is less stressful.

The following exhalation breath-hold protocols introduce minimally hypoxic conditions that will force the body to adapt to low levels of oxygen while you perform basic exercises. The balance in hypoxic training is creating short-term detrimental effects in order to achieve long-term adaptations that improve performance through greater endurance, improved recovery, and mental clarity. Pushing these exercises too aggressively can lead to maladaptations such as overload stress and anxiety and hinder achieving positive long-term effects.

These protocols use nasal breathing only, which helps the body manage itself and adapt to stress. Nasal breathing also promotes improved breathing mechanics and oxygenation. As you did in the Buteyko method, after each set of exhale holds, stop and fully recover before starting another set. Full recovery will prevent triggering a stress response that creates anxiety.

To perform the exhale breath-hold protocols, breathe through the nose to calm the body and nervous system. After the final exhalation, perform the movement while holding your breath. Recover by breathing through the nose until breathing returns to normal. On average, it takes 5 to 10 breaths through the nose or 15 to 30 seconds to recover. After full recovery, exhale and do the movement again. If you must take the first few recovery breaths through the mouth, you held your breath too long. The exercise should be done with only nasal breathing throughout.

Intermittent Hypoxic Training

Intermittent hypoxic training (IHT) simulates high-altitude training and is a great way to simulate training high and living low, a practice many professional athletes follow. The key word is *intermittent*. Training with lower levels of oxygen is not meant to be sustained for a long time. The body is not meant to function in hypoxic situations. When used properly, minimal doses of hypoxic training provide significant adaptations and increase oxygen-carrying capacity. IHT can improve aerobic capacity and oxygen use in muscle tissue and can improve focus and energy that can be used immediately in performance. If you're feeling tired or lack focus, it may be useful to use one of the exhale breath-hold protocols on pages 104 to 105 to create a hypoxic (low oxygen) condition. This will produce a small amount of extra red blood cells and oxygenated muscle tissue that may optimize performance in the moment. Use three to five rounds of exhale holds with movement before performing. This exercise will not provide long-term benefits, but acute exposure to stress on the cells of the body can enhance performance in the moment.

Endurance Breath Holds With Endurance Exercises

The protocols in this section are used in conjunction with endurance exercises and are great for warming up and activating the system before training and competition. When using them to warm up, stick to either walking or jogging. Breath holding during sprints should be used in training environments, specifically at the start of an aerobic training session. If you use them before competition, cut the time or reps in half and perform only one exercise. You can pick one of the three exercises in this section and focus solely on it or combine exercises by cutting the times and reps in thirds and performing them in this order: walk, jog, sprint.

Walk

Walk with consistently timed steps and breathe through the nose only for 15 to 30 seconds. Exhale and hold your breath while you continue to walk. Once you feel a strong need to breathe, breathe through the nose to recover and continue walking during the recovery period. Once you are breathing normally again, exhale and repeat. Perform this exercise for 10 minutes.

Jog

Jog with consistently timed steps and breathe through the nose only for 15 to 30 seconds. Exhale and hold your breath while you continue to jog. Once you feel a strong need to breathe, breathe through the nose to recover and continue jogging during the recovery period. Once you are breathing normally again, exhale and repeat. Perform this exercise for 10 minutes.

Sprint

Stand still and breathe through the nose for 15 to 30 seconds. When ready, exhale, hold the breath, and sprint as far as you can until you feel a strong need to breathe. Stop and breathe through the nose to recover. You will remain stopped in the recovery phase of this exercise. Once you have recovered completely and are breathing normally, exhale and repeat. Perform 10 sprints, trying to cover the same distance each time.

Exhale Breath Holds With Agility Exercises

The protocols in this section are used in conjunction with endurance and agility exercises and are great for warming up and activating the system before training and competition. When using them to warm up, perform the one you find most enjoyable. Breath holding during agility exercise should be used in training environments, specifically at the start of an aerobic session. If you use them before competition, cut the time or reps in half and perform just one exercise. You can focus solely on one exercise or combine the two exercises by cutting the reps in half and performing them in this order: jump rope, high knees.

Jump Rope

Stand still and breathe through the nose for 15 to 30 seconds. When ready, exhale, hold your breath, and jump rope as fast as you can while counting your reps. When you feel a strong need to breathe, stop jumping, and breathe through the nose to recover. You will stop for each recovery phase. Once you feel you have recovered completely and are breathing normally, exhale and repeat. Perform 10 sets, trying to complete the same number of jumps each time.

High Knees

Stand still and breathe through the nose for 15 to 30 seconds. When ready, exhale, hold your breath, and perform high knees as fast as you can while counting your reps. When you feel a strong need to breathe, stop the exercise, and breathe through the nose to recover. You will stop for each recovery phase. Once you feel you have completely recovered and are breathing normally, exhale and repeat. Perform 10 sets, trying to complete the same number of reps each time.

Exhale Breath Holds With Strength Exercises

The protocols in this section are used in conjunction with endurance and strength exercises and are great for warming up and activating the system before training and competition. When using them to warm up, use the one you find most enjoyable. Breath holding during strength exercise should be used in training environments, specifically at the start of an aerobic session. If you use them before competition, cut the times and reps in half and perform just one exercise. You can focus solely on one exercise or combine exercises by cutting the times and reps in half and performing them in this order: farmer's carry, sled push.

Farmer's Carry

Stand with two kettlebells or dumbbells on the ground on either side of you and breathe through the nose for 15 to 30 seconds. Use a weight you can control and lower safely after the breath hold. When ready, exhale, hold your breath, pick up the weights, and walk as far as you can until you feel a strong need to breathe. Lower the weights slowly at your sides and breathe through the nose to recover. You will stop for each recovery phase. Once you feel you are fully recovered and are breathing normally, exhale and repeat. Perform 6 to 10 times, trying to cover the same distance each time.

Sled Push

Stand in front of an agility sled and breathe through the nose for 15 to 30 seconds. Use a weight you can control and push safely as you breath hold. When ready, exhale, hold your breath, and push the sled as far as you can until you feel a strong need to breathe. Stop pushing, and breathe through your nose to recover. You will stop for each recovery phase. Once you feel you have fully recovered and are breathing normally, exhale and repeat. Perform 6 to 10 times, trying to cover the same distance each time.

Hypoventilation Training

Hypoventilation training uses either abnormally slow breathing or short, consistent breath holds in conjunction with activities such as running, cycling, rowing, and swimming. These are not long breath holds because holding the breath too long taxes the body and leads to early exhaustion. Hypoventilation protocols should be performed only during training and not in competition.

During hypoventilation training, carbon dioxide levels rise while oxygen levels drop. Dr. James Counsilman is a former collegiate and U.S. Olympic swimming coach who coached numerous athletes to gold medals and is considered by many to be the most innovative coach in U.S. swimming history. He developed a method in the 1970s that restricted breathing frequency to create hypoxic conditions for swimmers. A traditional execution of hypoventilation consisted of taking a breath, holding it for an amount of time or number of strokes, and then exhaling and repeating the process. Dr. Counsilman proposed breathing every five or more strokes instead of the traditional two or three strokes. This forced the body to adapt to lower levels of oxygen. You don't need to be a swimmer or free diver to reap the benefits of hypoventilation training. Simple dry-land protocols in which you hold your breath following an exhalation drop oxygen levels and produce an effective stress on the body that produces productive adaptation for performance.

Hypoventilation can be used three or four times a week in the off-season, which is often the time of the year when athletes try to push the body to extremes. During the season or recovery periods, perform hypoventilation once a week on aerobic days. This type of training doesn't cause serious health issues; however, it may be difficult, similar to any high-intensity training. If you have high blood pressure, cardiac disease, or pulmonary disease, you should consult with a medical professional before performing intense hypoventilation training protocols.

Pair your breathing with one of these movements to produce a drop in oxygen while training. If you can't breathe only through the nose for 10 to 15 minutes, start with 5 minutes and build up. The breath holds should not be long enough to stop the movement or disrupt the pace. If you feel the breath holds are too stressful, lower their frequency or the length of time you hold them, or move at a slower pace.

Run or Jog

Run or jog at a pace you can control and pace your steps with your breath, inhaling through the nose for three seconds (3 steps) and exhaling through the nose for three seconds (3 steps). After five or six breaths, complete a normal exhalation through the nose, and hold your breath while counting 10 steps (if you can hold your breath for only 6 or 8 steps that is fine; you can work up to 10). Inhale through the nose again for three seconds (3 steps) and exhale through the nose for three seconds (3 steps) for another five or six breaths. Continue the cycle for 10 to 15 minutes. You don't have to complete this exercise perfectly. The goal is performing exhale holds in rhythm with your pace and lowering the breath frequency while you run. This exercise requires mental focus.

Row Machine

Two movements occur in this exercise, and you will pace your breath with those movements. Inhale as you enter the starting position of the row, and exhale as you push with your legs and pull with your arms to complete the row. Perform five reps on the row, breathing normally through the nose. After five reps, hold after the fifth exhalation, and perform two more rows while holding your breath. Continue to row slowly in rhythm with your inhalations and exhalations as you gather your breath and reach full recovery. Once your breath returns to normal, repeat. Perform for 10 to 15 minutes.

Stationary Bike

While riding a stationary bike, inhale through the nose for 3 seconds and exhale through the nose for 3 seconds. After five total breaths, exhale through the nose and hold for 6 to 10 seconds. Once you've completed the hold, breathe normal and keep pedaling as you recover. Once your breathing has returned to normal and you feel recovered, repeat. Perform for 10 to 15 minutes.

Oxygen Therapy Chambers

Oxygen chambers have become popular in the athletic community. In hyperbaric oxygen therapy, athletes breathe 100 percent oxygen (the air we breathe is 21 percent oxygen) inside a chamber where the pressure has been raised higher than normal to help the lungs collect more oxygen. This helps tissues accumulate more oxygen and heal. Hypobaric chambers remove oxygen from the chamber to simulate high altitude. These chambers are used to reduce inflammation, help immune cells destroy bacteria, and simulate the formation of blood vessels, allowing areas of the body to improve oxygenation. The hyperbaric chamber counteracts low levels of oxygen in the body, which can lead to illness, injuries, and poor performance.

The biggest difficulty in using a hyperbaric or hypobaric chamber to oxygenate the body is access. Consistent use is required to reap long-term benefits from this type of therapy. Most athletes need treatments at least once a week and as many as five times a week. It may also take several weeks of consistency to find benefits.

You now have many exercises to build your capacity to hold your breath. Use these practices intentionally to not only improve your game but also to raise your awareness of yourself. As stated early in the chapter, be consistent. Apply both the static and moving breath-holding protocols to training and competition days as well as days off. Over time, concentrate less on the length of time you can hold your breath and focus more on how you feel when you hold your breath. A mountain remains strong and still through all weather conditions. Breath holding will always feel different, so regardless of what is going on around you, be the mountain.

7

Strengthening Exercises

As the muscles involved in breathing get stronger, lung capacity and levels of endurance will improve. By consciously building stronger muscles of respiration through the exercises in this chapter, you will be able to take fewer breaths both outside of and during performance, which helps sustain the balance of energy. In addition to improved lung health, you should also notice improvements in your mobility during training and competition. And you will build awareness of the movements that take place during respiration.

This chapter describes a variety of breathing techniques and range of exercises that help the body function properly so you can choose the exercises most suitable for you. Focusing on the breath during these protocols can take time to master and become comfortable with. Take your time learning the practices and finding those that fit you best.

The chapter starts with exhalation-strengthening practices that help you control your exhalation and build awareness of the muscles used in respiration. Chapter 5 described an exercise to measure the length of an exhalation. When your breathing muscles are strong enough to control the length of your exhalation, you will feel calmer, perform well under pressure, and improve your ability to remain healthy.

To improve your breathing skills, use horizontal and diaphragmatic breathing, and as you exhale, use your abdominal muscles to manage the pace and speed of exhalation. As you continue breathing practices, this will become easier. You can use the exhale test in chapter 5 on page 89 to track improvement.

Next, the chapter focuses on inhalation exercises, rib cage mobility, spine mobility, and the pelvic floor. It is important to use breathing exercises to keep these areas healthy. The pelvic floor, which was discussed in chapter 2, is the lowest breathing muscle and it moves with the thoracic diaphragm. Strengthening and controlling the pelvic floor not only helps the internal organs function properly, but protects the torso as well. If you want to warm up before these exercises, use the breathing warm-ups in chapter 5.

Exercises to Strengthen Exhalation Muscles

The following exercises strengthen the muscles involved in exhalation. The exhalation is a passive movement. As you exhale, the ribs move down and rotate in to help the diaphragm push the air out of the lungs, and the pelvic floor pushes up against the bottom of the organs to complete the exhalation phase of breathing. These exercises strengthen both the diaphragm and pelvic floor and the abdominal muscles, which are also crucial in supporting the expiration process. As the diaphragm pushes back up into the rib cage, you need the support of a strong abdominal wall to apply pressure to finalize a full exhalation.

Maximum Inhalation With Controlled Exhalations

In this exercise you will perform a maximum inhalation followed by a pursed-lip controlled exhalation. You will learn how to control your exhalation and how to properly expand the lungs. You will focus on expanding the rib cage and bringing in as much air as possible during the inhalation and then using the breathing muscles to push all the air out of the lungs in a controlled, slow exhalation.

Begin by sitting on the floor in a cross-legged position or in a chair with the feet flat on the ground. If you are unable to fully expand the lungs in these positions, lie faceup, with the knees bent and feet flat on the ground. In all positions, keep your arms at your sides or place one hand on your belly and the other hand on your chest. During the warm-up and working set of the protocol that follows, you will breathe in through the mouth in three stages. Imagine the inhalation as a wave that starts at your belly button and works its way up to your collarbone.

First, take a deep inhalation into the belly. Take a slight pause when you feel you have reached maximum capacity in your belly. Next, breathe into the lower and middle part of the rib cage as you expand around the middle of the sternum. Take a slight pause as you feel the middle of the chest opening. Finish the inhalation into the upper chest as you push the collarbones out and bring air into the top of the lungs. At the peak of this full inhalation, hold for one second and feel that your lungs are filled with air from top to bottom. Through pursed lips, begin the exhalation and make a quiet "whoosh" sound. Squeeze the abdomen muscles to help slow the pace of the exhalation. The focus on the exhalation is to slowly pull the belly button to the spine as you guide the diaphragm back under the ribs.

Here is the protocol for this exercise:

Warm-Up

Complete three full breaths performing the three-part inhalation process for each breath and then exhale for an increasing amount of time on each breath. Each inhalation should take about 10 seconds. The duration of the exhalation ensures you are able to fully control the exhalation after you have completely filled your lungs with air. The entire warm-up should take 90 seconds to two minutes.

- *Breath 1*: Inhale deeply through the mouth using the three-part inhalation, and then exhale through the mouth for at least 10 seconds.
- *Breath 2*: Inhale deeply through the mouth using the three-part inhalation, and then exhale through the mouth for at least 15 seconds.
- *Breath 3*: Inhale deeply through the mouth using the three-part inhalation, and then exhale through the mouth for at least 20 seconds.

Working Set

Once you can control a 20-second exhalation following a full inhalation, perform five more breaths, inhaling deeply through the mouth using the three-part inhalation and exhaling for 20 seconds. Again, the three-part inhalation takes about 10 seconds. As you improve, you can increase the time of the exhalation from 20 seconds to 30, 40, and up to 60 seconds.

Full-Exhalation Countdown

In this exercise you will completely exhale, and then train the residual volume of air in the lungs by counting down out loud. This strengthens the exhalation muscles.

Sit comfortably on the floor cross-legged or in a chair with your feet flat on the ground. Your spine is in a neutral position. A lying position is not recommended for this exercise. To begin, take a full inhalation through the nose (see figure *a*); you don't have to reach maximum capacity. After the inhalation, blow out all the air through the mouth (see figure *b*). When you feel there is no more air to exhale, squeeze the abdominal muscles to create tension and count down quietly (see figure *c*). The goal is to count as slowly as possible while holding the core tight and no air in the lungs. Take three breaths as follows:

- *Breath 1*: Inhale through the nose, exhale all air through the mouth, squeeze the abdominal muscles, and then count down from 10.
- *Breath 2*: Inhale through the nose, exhale all air through the mouth, squeeze the abdominal muscles, and then count down from 20.
- *Breath 3*: Inhale through the nose, exhale all air through the mouth, squeeze the abdominal muscles, and then count down from 30.

After the countdown, focus on taking a calm and deep inhalation through the nose. Once you can easily count down from 30, increase the number, but keep in mind that you should be able to take a controlled inhalation after each count-down. If you can't count down slowly or take a controlled inhalation afterward, the number is too high.

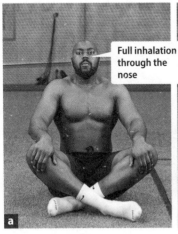
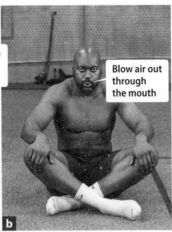
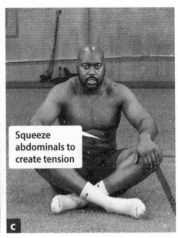

Balloon Exhalation Series

This group of exercises uses a balloon to help you lengthen your breath, strengthen your exhalation muscles, and build breathing strength. The balloon helps you breathe all the air out while maintaining a relaxed jaw. If using the balloon is too difficult, you can perform the exercises without a balloon, but first try them all with a balloon. Also, before you start, stretch the balloon to make it easier to blow air into it. You may also want to blow a little air into the balloon to make it easier to blow up when exhaling.

Chest Expansion Breath

The objective of this exercise is to expand the rib cage and create length from the bottom of the ribs to the hip bones. Because the front of the ribs will expand and create space for the muscles between each rib, the exhalation will be used to strengthen the abdominal muscles involved in exhalation. To begin, sit either on the ground in a cross-legged position or in a chair with the feet flat on the floor. Maintain a tall spine. You will use mouth breathing only throughout this exercise. Take a deep inhalation through the mouth, lengthening the spine and expanding the front of the ribs as much as possible (see figure *a*). Pull the shoulder blades back at the peak of inhalation to create expansion across the upper chest above the nipples. The head is tilted up slightly.

As you reach the peak of the inhalation, put the balloon in your mouth and exhale through the mouth into the balloon while bringing the chin down toward the chest and push the shoulder blades into a forward position. Focus on exhaling while pulling the belly button in toward the spine to cave the body forward, and pushing all the air out into the balloon (see figure *b*). Perform two sets of 15 breaths.

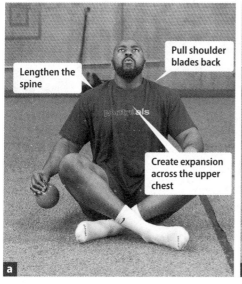
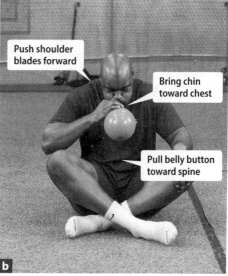

Monkey Hang Breath

The objective of this exercise is to create length in the body by hanging from a pull-up bar. The inhalation will lengthen the rib cage. When you are exhaling, you should feel your rib cage being pulled down and your pelvic floor being engaged. Your legs may come forward, but the spine stays neutral as you exhale. This is the result of pelvic floor activation.

   To begin, hang from a pull-up bar with the palms facing away from the body and with a balloon in the mouth. Take a bigger than normal breath in through the nose until you feel you have reached peak inhalation (see figure *a*), and then exhale the air slowly through the mouth into the balloon. Bring the chin down slightly and pull up the pelvic floor as you begin the exhalation (see figure *b*). This will connect the center of the body and help you control the exhalation. This exercise requires grip strength and a controlled breath to keep the spine neutral. Perform two sets of five breaths.

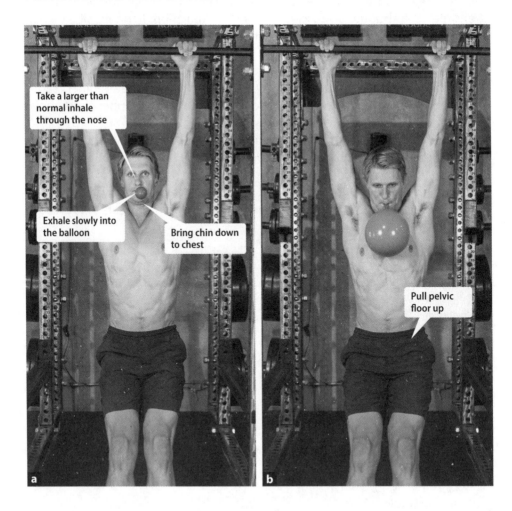

Lying V-Up Breath

The objective of this exercise is to strengthen the abdominal muscles involved in breathing as well as engage the pelvic floor on exhalation. Lie faceup and press the rib cage down so the lower back is on the ground. Hold a balloon in one hand. Take an inhalation through the nose and bring the balloon to the mouth (see figure *a*). As you begin exhaling, perform a V-up and exhale into the balloon (see figure *b*). Keep the lower back on the ground the entire time. Perform two sets of five breaths.

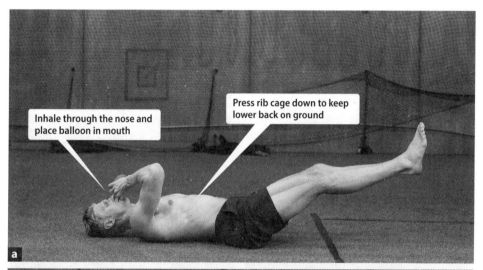

Inhale through the nose and place balloon in mouth

Press rib cage down to keep lower back on ground

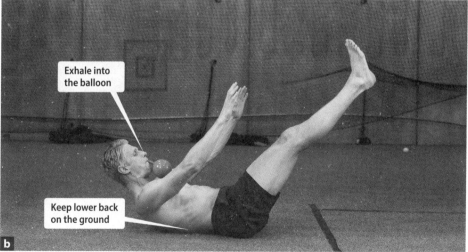

Exhale into the balloon

Keep lower back on the ground

90-90 Wall Breath

The objective of this exercise is to strengthen the abdominal muscles and dia-phragm while keeping the spine in a neutral position. To begin, lie faceup with the hips and knees at 90-degree angles and the feet flat against a wall. Press the rib cage down so the lower back is on the ground. Lift the hips so you're about one inch (2.5 centimeters) off the ground to activate the hamstrings. Place one hand on your belly, and hold the balloon with the other. Take a big inhalation through the nose, feeling the air in the belly and then the chest. Once you feel the breath has reached the chest and the rib cage, put the balloon in your mouth (see figure *a*). Exhale through the mouth into the balloon while pushing the rib cage down into the ground (see figure *b*). This will put the pelvis in a neutral position and activate the abdominal muscles. Perform two sets of five breaths.

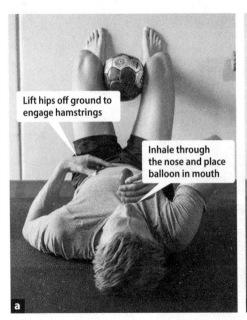

Lift hips off ground to engage hamstrings

Inhale through the nose and place balloon in mouth

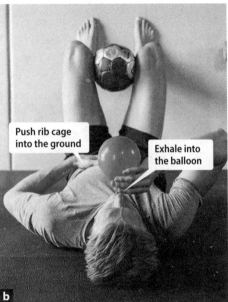

Push rib cage into the ground

Exhale into the balloon

Standing Breath

The objective of this exercise is to strengthen the abdominal muscles and create length in the body. This is similar to the chest expansion breath, except you're standing while performing the exercise. To begin, stand tall with the feet hip-width apart. Hold the balloon in your dominant hand. Take a bigger than normal breath in through the nose while lengthening the spine and lifting the head and chin slightly (see figure *a*). Bring your shoulder blades back at the peak of inhalation to expand the upper chest, and place the balloon in your mouth at the end of the inhalation. Slowly exhale into the balloon as long as possible as you bring the chin in toward the chest, squeezing your abdominal muscles as you exhale (see figure *b*). You should feel the rib cage being pulled down. This breath will be complete as you finish in a neutral position, with the ribs directly over the hips and a filled balloon. Perform two sets of 10 breaths.

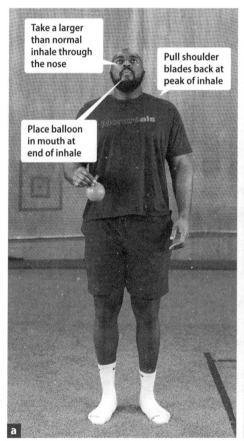
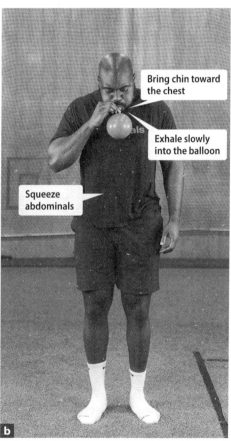

Fast-Twitch Activation Breathing

These breathing exercises strengthen the abdominal muscles and help you control the pelvic floor while breathing faster. If these exercises cause you to feel light-headed or dizzy, reset and breathe through the nose until the symptoms subside. Fast breathing can create a feeling of energy and focus afterward.

Bellow Breath

The objective of this exercise is to breathe as fast as possible on both the inhalation and the exhalation. To begin, sit comfortably on the floor in a cross-legged position. You can sit on a pillow to lift the hips. Place both hands at the bottom and side of your ribs (see figure). Place the tongue at the roof of the mouth and take 10 nasal breaths as fast and deep as possible. On the 11th breath, inhale through the nose as deep as you can and hold it for 10 to 15 seconds, then exhale as slowly as you can through the nose. Perform three sets.

Next, take 30 short and sharp nasal breaths, using the abdominal muscles to squeeze the breath out. After 30 breaths, take a deep inhalation through the nose and hold for 10 to 15 seconds, then exhale as slowly as you can through the nose. Perform three sets of 30 exhalations.

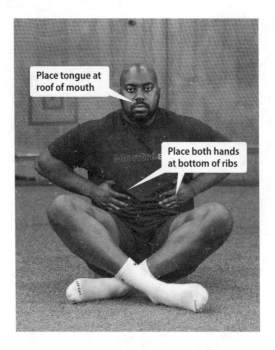

Breath of Fire

This exercise is a form of kundalini yoga breathing, which involves passive inhalation and aggressive exhalation. In yoga, the purpose of this breathing practice is to release toxins and chemicals from the cells in the body. You can use this practice to expand your lung capacity and strengthen the abdominal muscles. During a normal inhalation, push the belly out, and then during the exhalation, aggressively pull the belly button in toward your spine and force the air out quickly.

To perform this exercise, sit tall either in a cross-legged position on the floor or in a chair with your feet flat on the floor. Place both hands over the belly button. Inhale and exhale through the nose in quick succession; the inhalation happens almost automatically through the nose, and you make a sound as you quickly and forcefully exhale through the nose. As you inhale, press the belly out into your hands (see figure *a*), and as you exhale, pull the belly button into the spine (see figure *b*). Perform two sets of 50 breaths.

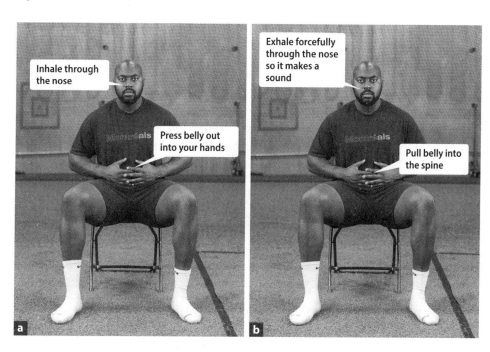

Candle Blowout Breath

The objective of this exercise is to strengthen the abdominal muscles and control exhalation. Sit tall either on the floor in a cross-legged position or in a chair with the feet flat on the ground. Take a full inhalation through the nose while lengthening the spine, then exhale through pursed lips, trying to push all the air out of the lungs. Once you feel like all the air is out of the lungs, squeeze the abdominal muscles and hold your breath for one second. Following the breath hold, try to blow more air out of the lungs through the mouth as if you're blowing out a candle. Perform two sets of five breaths.

Exercises to Strengthen Inhalation Muscles

The following exercises strengthen the muscles involved in inhalation. Inhalation is primarily driven by the thoracic diaphragm, which separates the chest cavity from the abdomen. The goal of these exercises is to help you fully use the diaphragm while creating a full range of motion around the torso.

Partner-Push Breathing

In this exercise you will experience tension against the intercostals and diaphragm when inhaling. To perform the exercise, lie faceup on the floor, with the legs straight and arms by your side. A partner places their hands on the sides of your torso just below the nipples and cups the rib cage with the fingers down and thumbs on top. Breathing only through the nose, exhale most of your air out while your partner guides your ribs down. Take a five-second nasal inhalation while your partner applies light pressure against your rib cage as it expands (see figure a). Hold your breath for one second at the end of the inhalation, and then exhale while your partner pushes gently to guide the rib cage back down and in (see figure b). The pressure should not be strong enough to keep you from taking a five-second nasal inhalation. The pressure should be sufficient to create resistance for the diaphragm as it expands the rib cage 360 degrees. Your partner counts both the five-second inhalation and exhalation. Follow the cadence while breathing into your partner's pressure and back out. Perform one set of 10 breaths.

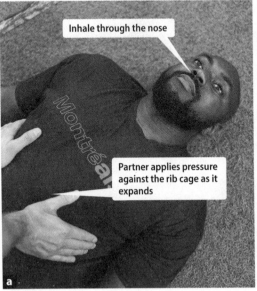
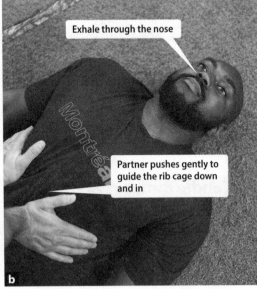

Banded-Pressure Breathing

This exercise is similar to the partner-push breathing, except the pressure comes from a band around the torso. The objective remains the same—to apply pressure around the rib cage, forcing the diaphragm to expand horizontally and against tension. To begin, sit crossed-legged on the floor, sit on a chair with the feet flat on the floor, or stand with the feet hip-width apart. Loop a resistance band around the bottom of the ribs, and pull each end with your hands to create tension.

To perform this exercise, exhale most of the air out of the lungs through the nose and at the same time, pull on the ends of the band to maintain tension and guide the ribs down and in. Next, take a deep inhalation through the nose and loosen the tension on the band while breathing horizontally into it (see figure *a*). The breath should expand the ribs 360 degrees and should fully use the diaphragm. Make sure the entire band maintains contact with the body while inhaling. Imagine you are a beverage can and you're filling yourself up with air from the inside. At the end of each inhalation, hold for one second. You should feel as if the rib cage is expanded 360 degrees, and the beverage can is filled completely with air.

After the inhalation, exhale through the nose while pulling the band gently to guide the ribs back down and in (see figure *b*). After a complete exhalation, pause for one second and take another deep inhalation through the nose, repeating the cycle. The inhalation should fill the rib cage area with air while the band provides tension. Perform one set of 10 breaths.

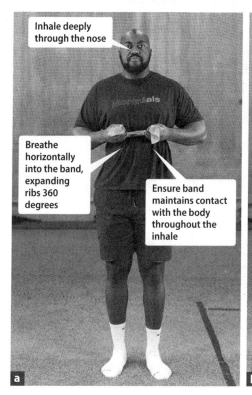

Inhale deeply through the nose

Breathe horizontally into the band, expanding ribs 360 degrees

Ensure band maintains contact with the body throughout the inhale

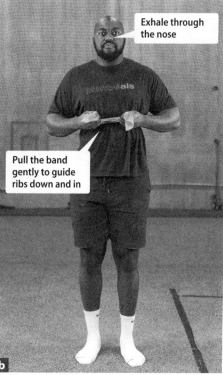

Exhale through the nose

Pull the band gently to guide ribs down and in

a
b

Rib Cage Pinch Breathing

The objective of this exercise is to feel your ribs moving on each inhalation and exhalation as well as to create tension around the ribs, which will force horizontal movement and a full range of motion of the diaphragm. To begin, sit tall in a chair with the feet flat on the ground or stand tall with the feet hip-width apart. With each hand, take your index fingers to your nipples and drag your hands straight down to your bottom ribs. Leave the index fingers on the bottom rib on each side while you wrap your thumbs around the back of your ribs. The index finger and thumb should have a good grip on the rib cage. Inhale deeply through the nose for four seconds. At the end of the inhalation, hold for one second. Exhale through the nose for eight seconds. Feel the rib cage move out and up on the inhalation (see figure *a*) and down and in on the exhalation (see figure *b*). Perform two sets of 20 breaths.

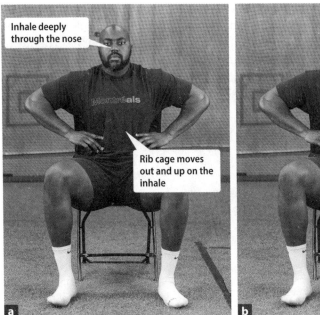
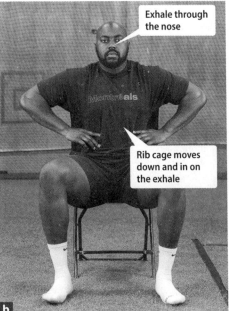

Counting Breath

The objective of this exercise is to expand the rib cage with small continuous inhalations, each followed by a pause, forcing you to control the diaphragm. To begin, sit tall either cross-legged on the floor or in a chair with the feet flat on the ground. Take a small breath in through the nose and pause, continuing the inhalations and pauses for five individual inhalations. Each inhalation will cause the rib cage to expand a little more. After you have completed five inhalations, finish the series with an exhalation through the nose, then repeat. Perform two sets of five inhalations. Once you can easily take five individual inhalations followed by one exhalation, increase the number of inhalations.

Exercises for Rib Cage, Spine, Back, and Pelvic Floor

The rib cage protects the internal organs, and the spine continually receives signals about your breathing patterns and efficiency. The pelvic floor works with the diaphragm to regulate pressure from inside the abdomen while supporting the spine. The following exercises will strengthen these areas of the body as well as improve mobility and flexibility throughout the body by creating space for the breathing muscles to expand and move freely.

Breathing properly and using these exercises to strengthen your breathing will help you avoid poor body positioning during training and competition. These exercises will be done in a supine position (lying faceup). This helps you to keep a healthy spine position, further access the diaphragm, and start engaging the pelvic floor. Follow the descriptions and try each of the practices to discover the one that works best for you and implement it into your training.

Supine Position Breathing

Although supine breathing exercises are staples for a healthy rib cage and spine, the thoracic diaphragm and pelvic floor breathing muscles are the primary focus. These exercises help you learn how to feel the pelvic floor moving and promote deep diaphragmatic breathing. The exercises are performed in three positions so you can feel how your body responds in different positions. It may help to have a towel or small pillow under your head to support the spine and relax the neck.

Supine Breathing

Lie faceup with your arms at your sides. Focus on bringing the rib cage down so the lower back is on the ground and you're able to maintain a healthy spine position (see figure). The shoulders are relaxed and should not be lifted toward your head. Keeping the spine neutral, slowly inhale through your nose for six seconds, expanding the rib cage to the sides, the front, and the back. The front of the rib cage will expand on the inhalation while you feel the back of the rib cage pushing into the ground. At the end of the inhalation, hold for four seconds. Then slowly exhale for eight seconds, pulling the front of the rib cage down as you keep the midback on the ground and engage the abdominal muscles. At the end of the exhalation, hold for four seconds. Repeat this sequence four times.

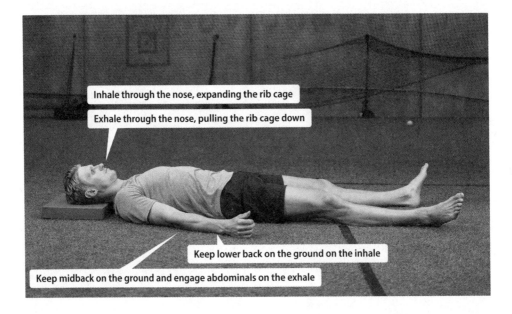

Supine Hook-Lying Breathing

This is a Postural Restoration Institute (PRI) breathing technique. Lie on your back with your knees bent and feet placed on a two-inch (5 centimeter) box or block. The block helps you posteriorly rotate the pelvis, so your low back is against the floor, which will help you activate the hamstrings and glutes instead of the low back during the movement. Place a resistance band around your legs just above the knees. Your arms are at your sides and your elbows bent 90 degrees so your hands are in the air. Start with your knees together and inhale through your nose as you open your knees and move your hands out to the side while keeping your elbows stationary. Take a full inhalation that lasts as long as the movement of the knees and hands (see figure *a*). Exhale through pursed lips as you slowly bring your knees and hands back together. At the end of exhalation, tilt the pelvis so that your tailbone is raised slightly off the ground while keeping your back flat on the ground (see figure *b*). The goal is to bring the bottom ribs closer to the front of the hips and returning to the original position with each breath. Concentrate on filling your chest more with each inhalation, using your diaphragm, keeping your neck relaxed, and achieving 360 degrees of rib cage expansion. Relax and repeat this sequence four more times, continuing the sequence of inhalation while lowering your hands and knees and then exhaling while bringing your hands and knees in, with a pelvic tilt at the end of each exhalation.

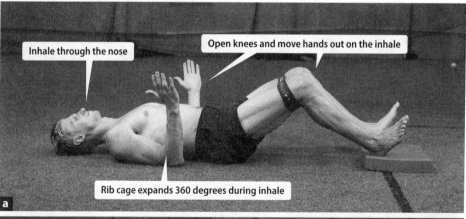

Inhale through the nose

Open knees and move hands out on the inhale

Rib cage expands 360 degrees during inhale

a

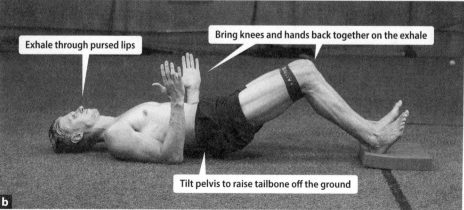

Exhale through pursed lips

Bring knees and hands back together on the exhale

Tilt pelvis to raise tailbone off the ground

b

Supine 90-90 Breathing

Lie faceup with your feet on a chair in a 90-90 position (hips and knees at 90-degree angles). Slightly lift the tailbone so that your back remains on the floor, and dig your heels into the chair to engage the hamstrings (see figure). Hold a soft ball, block, or towel between your knees to help you stay in position during the exercise. Inhale deeply through the nose for four seconds, expanding the rib cage to the sides, front, and back. At the end of the inhalation take a brief pause, then exhale through the mouth or nose for eight seconds, drawing the ribs down. At the end of the exhalation, hold another brief pause. Repeat this sequence four more times.

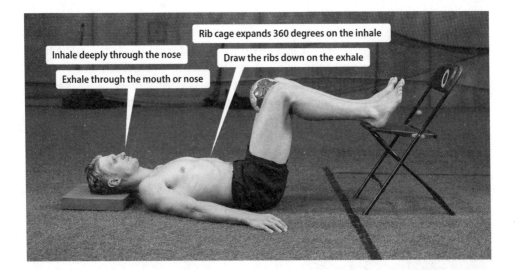

Intercostal Bends

The objective of this exercise is to create a stretch in the intercostal muscles and lengthen the rib cage. Sit tall in a chair with the feet flat on the ground. Keeping the head balanced and face straight ahead, reach one arm overhead. This keeps the spine tall. Inhale deeper than normal through the nose while reaching your middle finger higher into the air (see figure *a*). This should lengthen the intercostal muscles. As you reach a full inhalation, hold your breath and slightly bend to the side opposite the raised arm (see figure *b*). As you're bending, use that middle finger to guide the lengthening of the intercostals. After holding the breath and stretching to one side, bring the body back to the starting position as you exhale through the nose and relax the intercostals (see figure *c*). Perform two sets of five breaths on each side.

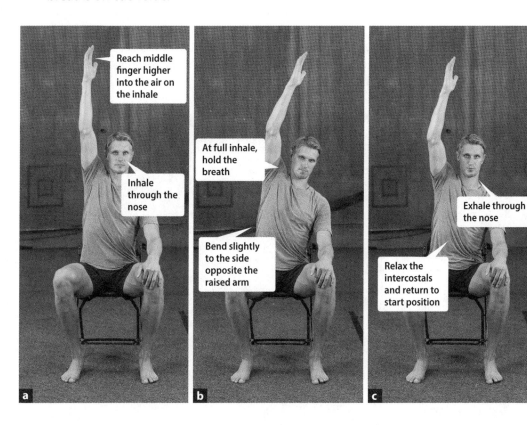

Standing Chest Expansion

The objective of this exercise is the same as a chest expansion breath presented earlier in this chapter. The goal remains expanding the chest and creating separation between the lower ribs and the top of the hips during an inhalation, and then bringing the ribs back over the hips and using the abdominal muscles to force air out during the exhalation. The standing position allows for more lengthening of the spine.

To start, stand tall with feet shoulder-width apart and pointing forward, and place the hands on the hips. Inhale deeply through the nose, pulling the elbows back to bring your shoulder blades closer together and open the chest (see figure *a*). At the same time, lengthen the spine as the chest begins to expand. Slightly lift the head and chin as you reach the top of the inhalation. Exhale slowly through the mouth as you bring the elbows back to the starting position, and bring your rib cage back over the hips as you use your abdominal muscles to squeeze the air out of the body (see figure *b*). Instead of trying to breathe for a certain amount of time, focus on reaching a peak inhalation, and exhale until you feel you have squeezed out all the air. Perform two sets of five breaths.

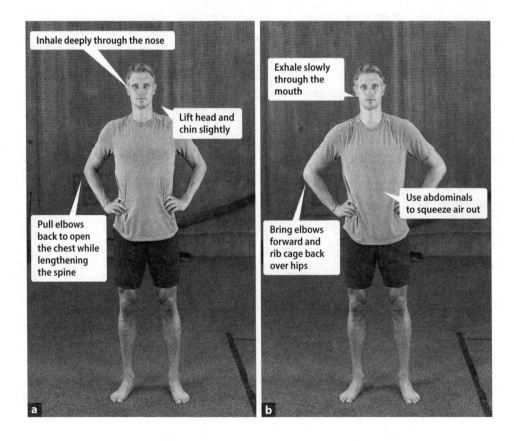

Hands-Behind-Head Chest Expansion

The objective of this exercise is to expand the chest, lengthen the spine, and open the rib cage. Sit tall either on the floor with legs crossed or in a chair with the feet flat on the ground. Interlock your fingers behind your head with your elbows out. Inhale deeply through the nose as you pull the elbows back, which will expand the chest and lengthen the spine (see figure *a*). You should feel like you are creating separation between the bottom ribs and the hip bones and that the front of the rib cage is expanding. As you reach the top of the inhalation, hold your breath for one second. Exhale slowly through pursed lips as you slowly bring the elbows back in toward the front of the body, caving your body inward (see figure *b*). At the same time, pull up the pelvic floor on the exhalation while you bring the belly button in toward the spine. The elbows will eventually touch in front of the sternum as you make your body small. At the end of the exhalation, gently pull on the back of the head and stretch the neck for one or two seconds. Once you've emptied all the air, start the deep inhalation through the nose again as you bring your body back into an extended and lengthened position with the elbows pulled back and the chest expanded. Perform two sets of five breaths.

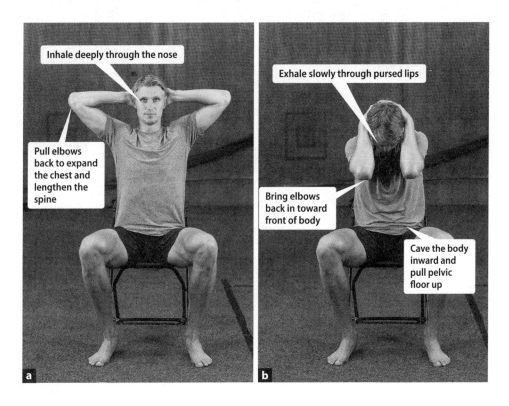

Cat–Cow Breathing

This exercise creates fluidity in the breath as it matches the movement between two positions—cat and cow. Get onto all fours with your shoulders over your wrists and your hips over your knees. The first movement is the traditional cow position from yoga. Inhale through the nose as you curve your lower back and lower the belly, roll the shoulders back, and lift your gaze toward the sky (see figure *a*). The next movement is the traditional cat. Exhale through the nose and reverse your position by arching the back upward, pulling the belly in while pushing the rib cage up, and looking in toward the navel (see figure *b*). Repeat the movement as you inhale and exhale. Perform two sets of 10 breaths.

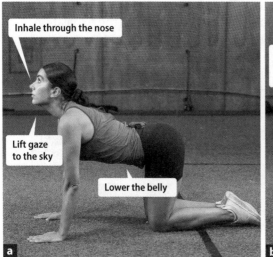
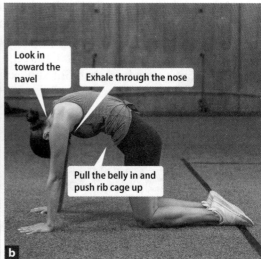

Dead Bug Breathing

The objective of this exercise is to strengthen the core, improve stability, and minimize pressure in the lower back by maintaining horizontal breathing, 360 degrees of rib cage expansion, and a full range of diaphragmatic movement. Lie on your back with the arms extended straight over the chest and perpendicular to the torso. With the hips and knees bent to 90 degrees, lift the feet off the ground (see figure *a*). Engage your core while your back maintains constant contact with the ground. The spine stays in this position throughout the exercise. Inhale through the nose, reaching your right arm back over your head and toward the floor while simultaneously extending your left knee and hip and reaching your left heel toward the floor (see figure *b*). The left arm and right leg don't move. Stop the movement just before the arm and foot touch the floor. Exhale through the nose and reverse the movement, returning the right arm and left leg to the start position (see figure *c*). Perform two sets of 20 breaths on each side (40 total).

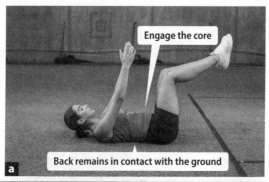

Engage the core

Back remains in contact with the ground

a

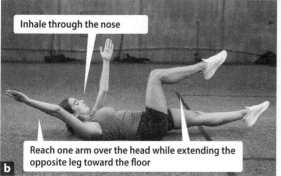

Inhale through the nose

Reach one arm over the head while extending the opposite leg toward the floor

b

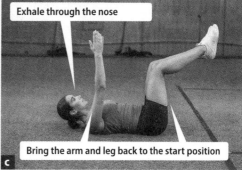

Exhale through the nose

Bring the arm and leg back to the start position

c

Child Pose Breathing

The objective of this exercise is to stretch the spine, thighs, hips, and ankles and to promote relaxation. Another benefit is breathing into the back ribs, which can be difficult. Kneel with your knees hip-width apart and lower your hips onto your heels while lowering your head to the ground and reaching your arms out into the traditional child's pose yoga position. If this hurts your knees, place them farther apart or place a pillow under your butt (see figure). You can also rest your head on a pillow if you can't reach the floor with the forehead. Inhale through the nose and fill the midsection cavity with air so you feel the belly pushing into your thighs and expanding through the waist and your back. Then exhale through the nose, letting the air out normally. You should feel relaxed in this position. Hold the position while breathing for 30 to 60 seconds.

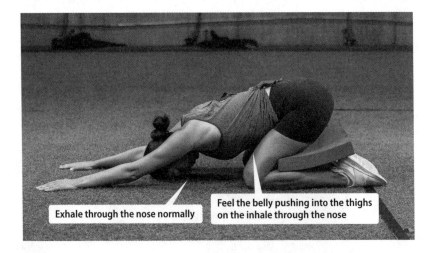

Exhale through the nose normally

Feel the belly pushing into the thighs on the inhale through the nose

Seated Spinal Twist Breathing

The objective of this exercise is to create a twist in the spine, which forces belly breathing that wrings out old air. The main cue in a spinal twist is to breathe deeply into the belly. By twisting around the spine and breathing deeply, you should feel a release in the lower back, hips, and groin. Sit tall either on the floor with legs crossed or on a chair with the feet flat on the ground. Inhale through the nose, reaching your left hand to the outer side of the right knee and your right arm behind your back or to the back of the chair (see figure). Hold the position gently as you finish the inhalation. While holding the position, exhale through the mouth and gently pull yourself deeper into the twist. Continue to hold the position following the exhalation and take three inhalations and exhalations to breathe deeper into the position while twisting the spine. You should feel tension around your spine and into your diaphragm. If it is painful, stop. Perform one full cycle on both sides.

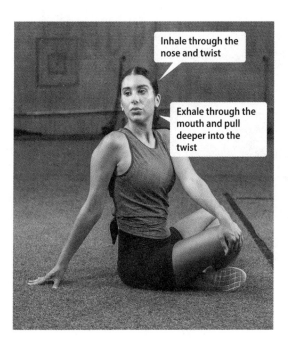

Side Plank Breathing

A side plank offers a variety of benefits: It strengthens the core, improves balance, and reduces the risk of a back injury. Holding a side plank and performing focused breathing helps you learn how to protect the spine. Use the side plank to not only gain strength but also to learn how to breathe horizontally and achieve 360-degree expansion while holding a plank. Lie on your right side with your legs straight and the top leg in front of the bottom leg for stability. Place your right elbow under your right shoulder with your forearm pointing away from you and your hand balled into a fist. The pinkie side should be in contact with the ground. The top arm can either be held in the air or positioned with the hand on the hip with a bent elbow to maintain balance. The head and neck should be in a neutral position. Lift the hips off the ground while keeping the body in a straight line from your bottom ankle to the top of your head (see figure). Breathe naturally in and out through the nose as you brace the core. Hold for 30 to 60 seconds on each side.

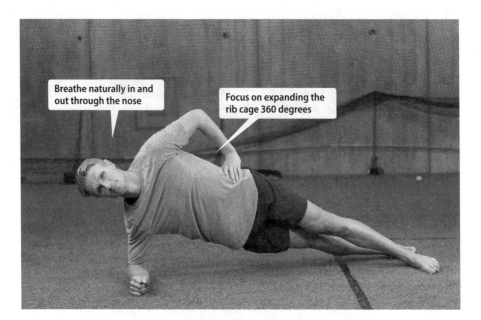

Crocodile Breathing

The objective of this exercise is to practice diaphragmatic breathing. While lying facedown, you will use the inhalation to push the belly into the ground, which forces the diaphragm to open the back ribs. This exercise also helps you eliminate shallow breathing. Lie facedown on the floor and rest your forehead on the hands (see figure). Inhale and exhale through the nose, using the belly to breathe into the ground so you feel the back lifting. The floor limits the direction of the movement of the belly during breathing, forcing the diaphragm to expand the lower back. Focus on taking slow and controlled inhalations for four to six seconds and hold a brief pause after the inhalation. Following the pause, slowly let the air out as you feel your belly button moving back toward the spine. The exhalation should be at least as long as the inhalation, but try to breathe out a second or two longer than you breathed in. Perform two sets of 10 breaths.

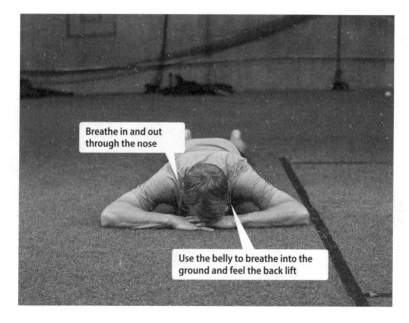

Stability Ball Back Breathing

This exercise helps you learn how to properly breathe into your back using horizontal, 360-degree breathing. Use the ball to apply pressure that will expand the back of the rib cage. Lie facedown on a stability ball with your forearms on the floor (see figure). If you are using a smaller stability ball, your knees can be on the ground. If you are using a bigger stability ball, your legs can be straight, with your toes pressed into the ground as shown. Keep the hips on the ball so you can't arch the back. Inhale through the nose and try to guide the air into the back. The pressure from the ball should help you feel your back ribs expanding. Visualize breathing into the upper ribs, then the middle ribs, and finally the bottom ribs. As you inhale, imagine creating space above and below each rib. Once you have taken a full inhalation, pause and then exhale through pursed lips. Try to inhale for at least four seconds and exhale for four to six seconds. Perform two sets of five breaths.

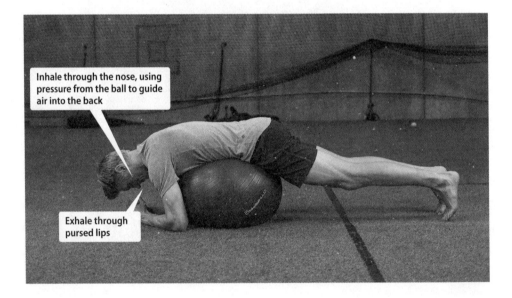

Inhale through the nose, using pressure from the ball to guide air into the back

Exhale through pursed lips

Deep-Squat Breathing

The objective of this exercise is to breathe in a natural position, force horizontal breathing and 360-degree expansion, and open the hips and groin. To start, sit in a deep squat with your back against a wall. You should be able to keep your heels on the ground and the knees slightly wider than shoulder width. Keep the arms inside the knees, and push against the knees with the elbows. If you cannot hold a deep squat, you will not be able to perform this exercise. Once in the squat position, lean forward so the belly is resting on the front of the quads, and the upper back, neck, and head are no longer against the wall. Take a deep inhalation through the nose into the belly while feeling the belly push into the top of the legs (see figure *a*). As you reach peak inhalation, pause briefly and exhale through pursed lips as the belly pulls back in toward the spine (see figure *b*). Perform two sets of five breaths.

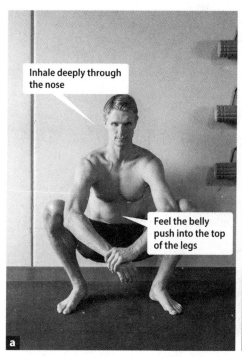
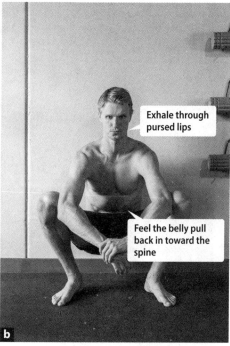

Lying Pelvic Floor Breathing

The objective of this exercise is to strengthen the pelvic floor muscles. Lie faceup with the knees bent and feet flat on the ground. Tilt the pelvis so the back is flat into the floor, and imagine that someone's hand is under the curve of your back. Inhale through the nose naturally as you slightly tilt your pelvis forward (see figure *a*), and then exhale through the nose gently while pushing the lower back into the ground as though you were pushing into the hand (see figure *b*). You shouldn't feel the leg muscles doing any of the work. This should all be done using the pelvis and lower core muscles. Perform two sets of 10 breaths.

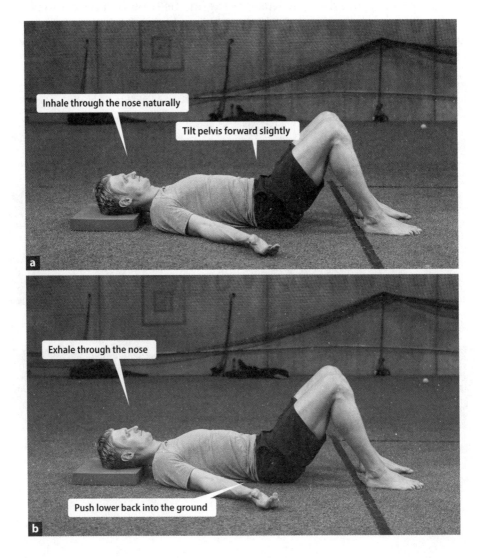

90-90 Lying Pelvic Floor Breathing

The objective of this exercise is to strengthen the pelvic floor muscles. While doing the breathing exercise, remember to breathe gently. Lie faceup with the feet on a sturdy chair, gently pushing the heels into the chair. Tilt the pelvis back so the back is flat into the floor, and imagine that someone's hand is under the curve of your back. Inhale through the nose naturally as you slightly tilt your pelvis forward (see figure *a*), and then exhale through the nose gently while pushing the lower back into the ground as though you were pushing into the hand (see figure *b*). You shouldn't feel the leg muscles doing any of the work. This should all be done using the pelvis and lower core muscles. Perform two sets of 10 breaths.

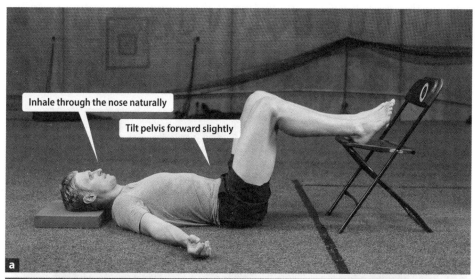

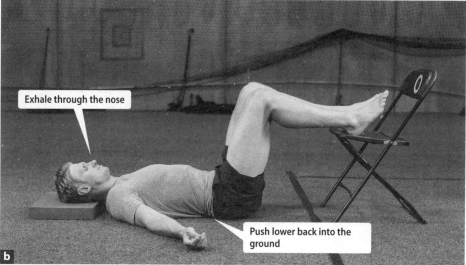

90-90 Pelvic Floor Breathing With Ball Between Knees

The objective of this exercise is to strengthen the pelvic floor muscles while maintaining control of a neutral spine. Hold a lightweight ball, such as a soccer ball or volleyball, between the knees, which are hip-width apart. Lie faceup, and raise the legs so that the hips and knees are bent to 90 degrees. You will not have a chair to stabilize the feet in this position. Keep the feet in the air. Tilt the pelvis back so the back is flat into the floor, and imagine that someone's hand is under the curve of your back. While squeezing the ball with the knees, inhale through the nose naturally (see figure *a*) and then exhale through the nose gently while pushing the lower back into the ground as though you were pushing into the hand (see figure *b*). Try to keep the leg muscles from doing the work; however, in this exercise with the feet in the air you may feel your glutes and hamstrings activated. Continue to focus on feeling your pelvis doing the work and feeling contraction in your lower core muscles. Perform two sets of 10 breaths.

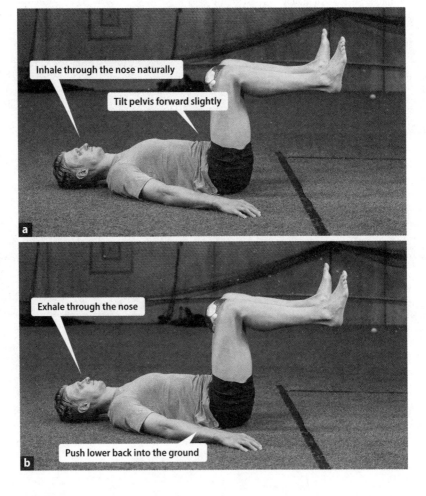

Single-Leg Lunge Pelvic Floor Breathing

The objective of this exercise is to strengthen the pelvic floor muscles as well as activating the glutes. To begin, assume a stationary lunge position, with the back knee on the ground while the front knee is directly over the front ankle. Keep the torso straight and core engaged while holding the position. Take a natural inhalation through the nose as you gently tilt the pelvis back (see figure *a*). You shouldn't move so much that the lower back is involved. This should be a gentle movement. Exhale through the nose or mouth twice as long as your inhalation as you squeeze the glutes and activate the pelvic muscles (see figure *b*). This will feel like the hip flexor is being stretched and the leg is firm. Pause for one or two seconds after the exhalation before inhaling again. Perform two sets of eight on each side.

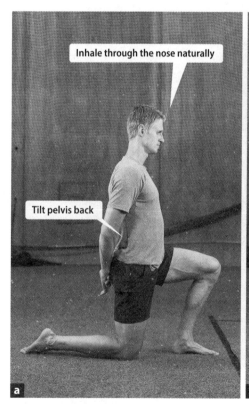

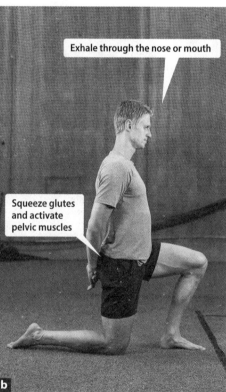

Monkey Hang Pelvic Floor Breathing

The objective of this exercise is to strengthen the pelvic floor muscles while hanging from a bar. This will require grip strength and body control to keep a neutral spine. Hang from a pull-up bar with palms facing away from the body (see figure). Inhale through the nose naturally as the spine lengthens. Exhale through the nose while pulling the ribs down and engaging the pelvic muscles to help push the air out. Exhale until you feel as though you have pushed all the air out. The pelvic muscles should control the spine so the body is not swaying and stays neutral. Breathe normally while performing two sets of five breaths.

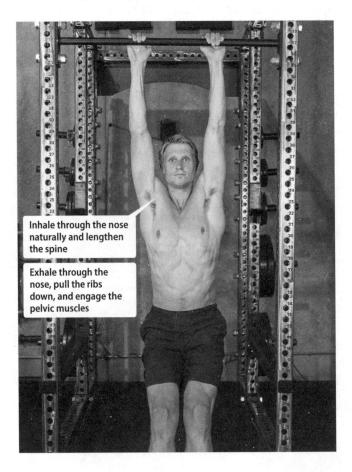

Inhale through the nose naturally and lengthen the spine

Exhale through the nose, pull the ribs down, and engage the pelvic muscles

Natural Movement Breathing

This exercise challenges you to put all the skills and strength developed through this chapter into use. The movement will require proper breathing and the ability to match the pace of the breath with the movement. It will provide a physical and mental challenge. Focus on maintaining horizontal movement of the diaphragm and 360 degrees of expansion while moving up and down from the floor. You will not be able to use your hands during this exercise, so you will need to protect the spine and keep the hips mobile while breathing properly.

During this exercise you will get up from the floor and back down to the floor without using your hands, using any movement you want, but there must be no delay in the movement. Begin seated on the ground in a cross-legged position with your hands gently resting on your feet (see figure *a*). From here, do whatever feels natural for you to get yourself off the floor without using your hands (see figures *b-c*). Inhale through the nose as you're starting the movement, exhale through the nose as you finish standing (see figure *d*). Inhale as you go back to the floor, exhale as you get back into a seated position. Breathing throughout the movements should be entirely through the nose. Complete 10 reps, then reverse the breathing and complete another 10 reps.

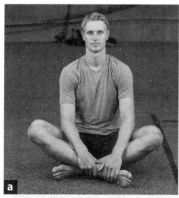
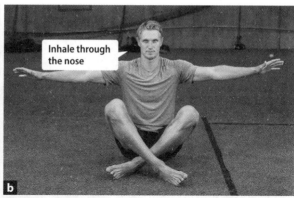
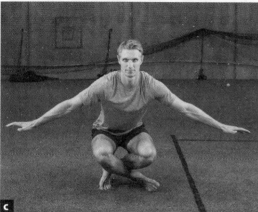
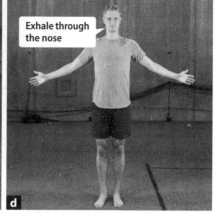

Your main focus in these breathing practices is to create movement with the breathing muscles that expands the rib cage 360 degrees. Any practice that moves the rib cage and expands the volume of the lungs is beneficial. Beyond expansion of the rib cage, you should be able to use your abdominal muscles and pelvic floor to complete exhalations. By strengthening these muscles, you will notice that your breathing becomes easier in training and competition. This will help you avoid overbreathing, using accessory muscles, and fatiguing. You should feel a natural rhythm with your breath and fluidity throughout the body while you're breathing. As the muscles of respiration get stronger, fluidity will happen unconsciously.

8

Recovery, Relaxation, and Emotional Regulation Exercises

The debate across the sport performance field is whether we should focus on high performance or injury prevention. Over the years, and especially in recent decades, we have seen incredible athletic feats. We run faster and jump higher while we have grown taller and stronger. But that has been accompanied by more injuries, anxieties, and pressures. This has created the need to balance where we place our attention. If we tip the balance toward being bigger, stronger, and faster, we are more likely to experience injury. As we work to maintain balance, we need to train hard, but recover even harder.

Today we have access to the most advanced environment of data-driven and science-based training. We have access to information and tracking devices that were unavailable to previous generations. The speed at which we can recover from injuries and surgeries has saved many careers. Scientists, coaches, and athletes search for ways to improve how we sleep, eat, train, and strategize. Breathing is the next push in advancing athletic potential. Breathing is the way to bridge the gap between high performance and high recovery.

The following are descriptions of recovery breathing exercises and guidelines for when to use them. The goal of the recovery process is to slow your breathing, which will trigger the parasympathetic nervous system to send oxygen to the muscles and to reset the nervous system before, during, and after training and competition. Your ability to clear your mind and open up space in your consciousness requires the same practice. Finding recovery breathing exercises that fit your needs will be a route of self-discovery.

Slowing the Breath Exercise

You will often find yourself breathing heavily in training or competition while your body is becoming fatigued or your thoughts becoming erratic. In these situations, you must understand the importance of slowing the breath by extending the exhalation to promote a parasympathetic state and proper breathing patterns. By dumping the air out in an extended exhalation, you will be ready for comfortable inhalations that expand the rib cage 360 degrees. If your breathing mechanics are sound, you will be successful in lowering the rate of respiration and calming both the body and the mind.

The goal is to achieve calm nasal breathing as you enter a recovery zone. When the breath is fast and through the mouth, chances are you are competing or training hard. Here is an example of down-regulating the breath when you are stressed. First, focus on controlling and becoming aware of your breath. Once you feel you have control of your breath, inhale through the nose followed by a natural pause. As the heart rate begins to slow and the breathing feels less stressed, try breathing entirely through the nose while focusing on a rhythmic pace. If your heart rate still feels too high and breathing through the nose is stressful, continue mouth breathing on both the inhalation and the exhalation until your body and breathing are calm enough to support total nasal breathing.

Here is a step-by-step process for slowly lowering the respiration rate and calming the system for recovery immediately following a performance or a training session:

1. Sit tall with a neutral spine either in a chair with the feet flat on the ground or cross-legged on the floor. If you feel more comfortable lying down, lie on your back with your arms at your sides or one hand resting on the belly and the other on the chest. The knees should be bent and the feet flat on the ground.

2. Breathe in and out through the mouth with a pause after the inhalation and an extended exhalation (five to nine sets).

3. Breathe in through the nose with a brief pause and out through the mouth with an extended exhalation (five to seven sets).

4. Breathe in through the nose with a brief pause and out through the nose (three to five sets). You can count this rhythmic breathing pace or feel it naturally. Try to maintain a cadence of three seconds for the inhalation with a natural pause and three seconds for the exhalation.

If your heart rate isn't too high and your focus is on the breath to create a state of mindfulness and calmness, you can skip the previous exercise and do the following to slow the mind and body:

1. Sit tall with a neutral spine either in a chair with the feet flat on the ground or cross-legged on the floor. If you feel more comfortable lying down, lie on your back with your arms at your sides or one hand resting on the belly and the other on the chest. The knees should be bent and the feet flat on the ground.

2. Place all of your attention on the breath and blow all the air out through the mouth making a "whoosh" sound.

3. Follow the exhalation with a slow and controlled inhalation through the nose. Pause at the top of the inhalation and release the air naturally and smoothly through the nose on the exhalation.

4. Repeat for three to five minutes.

EPOC Breathing

EPOC (excess post-oxygen consumption) breathing is a series of protocols for regulating your breathing in moments of recovery. During training, you may have just one to three minutes between sets or during breaks in competition to regulate the breath. Three levels of EPOC breathing protocols can be used for adaptation during these times. Which protocol you use depends on the intensity of your activity. Begin in one of three positions: standing with a neutral spine, seated on a chair with your feet flat on the ground, or lying faceup on the ground with the arms at your sides and palms facing up.

High Intensity

Use this protocol when you are working at high intensity. It will take you approximately three minutes to recover.

1. Breathe in through the mouth and out through the mouth for 60 seconds. Take a brief pause after each inhalation and exhalation.
2. Breathe in through the nose and out through the mouth for 60 seconds. Take a brief pause after each inhalation and exhalation.
3. Breathe in through the nose and out through the nose for 60 seconds. Take a brief pause after each inhalation and exhalation.
4. Finish by taking three breaths: four-second inhalation through the nose, pause, seven-second exhalation through the nose.

Moderate Intensity

Use this protocol when you are working at moderate intensity. It should take approximately two minutes to recover.

1. Breathe in through the nose and out through the mouth for 60 seconds. Take a brief pause after each inhalation and exhalation.
2. Breathe in through the nose and out through the nose for 60 seconds. Take a brief pause after each inhalation and exhalation.
3. Finish by taking three breaths: four-second inhalation through the nose, pause, seven-second exhalation through the nose.

Low Intensity

Use this protocol when you are working at low intensity. It will take about a minute to recover.

1. Breathe in through the nose and out through the nose for 60 seconds. Take a brief pause after each inhalation and exhalation.
2. Finish by taking three breaths: four-second inhalation through the nose, pause, seven-second exhalation through the nose.

EPOC is a concept to help you become aware that even when you're done training or competing, your engine is still running. By using the breath to slow down after training or competition, you accelerate the recovery process. After training or competition, take 10 to 30 minutes to regulate your breathing. The recovery practices in this chapter should be done immediately following training or competition. Over time you will learn which practice works best for you. Your goal is to bring the system back to neutral and adapt faster.

Coherent Breathing

Coherent breathing is slow, even, nasal breathing that devotes the same amount of time to the inhalation and exhalation, typically five seconds for each. This promotes positive psychological and physiological responses by breathing at a respiratory rate of six breaths per minute. Chronic sympathetic activity in the nervous system happens because of chronic overbreathing, which is breathing at a high respiration rate. By lengthening the breath cycle and creating coherent breathing patterns, you can alleviate the feelings associated with sympathetic activity. By slowing the rate of respiration, you can balance the nervous system. Coherent breathing is a mindful practice you can use any time and any place, and it complements the breath practices in this chapter. You can perform coherent breathing before or after any of the practices to keep yourself neutral. By first focusing on coherent breathing, you not only become mindful of your breath, but you also become aware of your body. Putting yourself in a neutral position both before and after breathing practices helps you develop mental and physical space.

Begin from one of these positions: stand tall, sit on a chair with the feet flat on the ground, sit cross-legged on the ground, or lie faceup on the floor. First, empty the lungs by blowing all your air out through the mouth. Take a slow inhalation through the nose for five seconds, briefly pausing after the inhalation. Exhale through the nose for five seconds, briefly pausing after the exhalation. Repeat for 10 minutes.

Cadence Breathing

Cadence breathing, like coherent breathing, is meant to create a consistent flow and rhythm in the breath. The inhalation and exhalation are the same length, with a natural pause after both. Use this exercise in the morning, before training or competition, or during the evening. This exercise can be done daily and even multiple times a day.

To begin, sit upright on a chair with the feet flat on the ground or sit cross-legged on the floor. Rest your arms at your sides, with your hands on your legs and the palms facing up. The palms do not need to face up if this is uncomfortable. This arm position pulls the shoulder blades back, which helps the rib cage expand. Maintain a tall posture and avoid hunching the shoulders forward. A posture that disrupts a neutral spine or inhibits diaphragmatic movement negatively affects breathing. The jaw should be relaxed, and the tongue should be pressed against the roof of the mouth just behind the top teeth.

Make sure you are able to do steps 1 and 2 before moving on to steps 3 and 4. You should be able to maintain at least 10 minutes of the first two steps without stress before adding time. The higher the cadence, the fewer breaths you will take. The goal of slow, cadence breathing is to reduce the number of breaths you take in a minute. These protocols should create calm and relaxing sensations.

1. Inhale through the nose for 3 seconds, pause, exhale through the nose for 3 seconds, and take a brief pause.
2. Inhale through the nose for 5 seconds, pause, exhale through the nose for 5 seconds, and take a brief pause.
3. Inhale through the nose for 7 seconds, pause, exhale through the nose for 7 seconds, and take a brief pause.
4. Inhale through the nose for 10 seconds, pause, exhale through the nose for 10 seconds, and take a brief pause.

Cadence Breathing With a Hold

Cadence breathing with a hold is the same as coherent breathing and cadence breathing in that it is meant to create a consistent flow and rhythm in the breath while focusing on controlling the exhalation with the diaphragm. The inhalation and exhalation are the same length, but instead of pausing after the inhalation, you hold for the same amount of time. This exercise slows the rate of respiration and forces you to control the exhalation with the abdominal muscles. You can perform this exercise daily and even multiple times a day.

To begin, sit upright either on a chair with the feet flat on the ground or cross-legged on the floor. The arms are at the sides with the palms facing up on top of the legs. The jaw is relaxed, and the tongue is pressed against the roof of the mouth just behind the top teeth.

Make sure you are able to do steps 1 and 2 before moving on to steps 3 and 4. You should be able to maintain at least 10 minutes of the first two steps without stress before adding time. The higher the cadence, the fewer breaths you will take. The goal of slow cadence breathing with a hold is to lower the number of breaths you take in a minute. These protocols should create calm and relaxing sensations.

1. Inhale through the nose for 3 seconds, hold for 3 seconds, then exhale through the nose for 3 seconds. Take a brief pause after the exhalation.

2. Inhale through the nose for 5 seconds, hold for 5 seconds, then exhale through the nose for 5 seconds. Take a brief pause after the exhalation.

3. Inhale through the nose for 7 seconds, hold for 7 seconds, then exhale through the nose for 7 seconds. Take a brief pause after the exhalation.

4. Inhale through the nose for 10 seconds, hold for 10 seconds, then exhale through the nose for 10 seconds. Take a brief pause after the exhalation.

4-7-8 Breathing

The 4-7-8 protocol was developed by Andrew Weil, MD, a pioneer in the field of integrative health. The 4-7-8 breathing protocol, also known as the relaxing breath, is a simple, effective way to combat stress. The goal behind the breathing practice is to gain control of your breath. When it is practiced regularly, this technique can help people fall asleep faster. Use this exercise any time of day and as often as needed before or during breaks in training or competition to help you relax and reduce anxiety or after competition or training to promote recovery.

To begin, sit upright either on a chair with the feet flat on the floor or cross-legged on the ground. The arms should be resting at your sides and palms facing up on top of the legs. The jaw is relaxed, and the tongue is pressed against the roof of the mouth just behind the top teeth. To perform this exercise, completely exhale the air through the mouth while making a "whoosh" sound. Then close your mouth and inhale through the nose quietly for four seconds. Follow the nasal inhalation with a seven-second hold, then exhale completely through the mouth making a "whoosh" sound for eight seconds. This is considered one breath. Repeat the cycle three more times for a total of four breaths.

Box Breathing

Box breathing, also known as square breathing, is a practice to lower the number of breaths you take. Start by exhaling all the air through the mouth. Inhale, then hold the breath, exhale, and then hold the breath. The breaths and holds are the same length. For example, if the inhalation is four seconds, the holds and exhalation will also be four seconds. It is referred to as box breathing because a box has four sides. Use this exercise any time of day and as often as needed before or during breaks in training or competition to help you relax and reduce anxiety or after competition or training to promote recovery.

To begin, sit upright on a chair with the feet flat on the floor or cross-legged on the ground. The arms are resting at the sides, with your palms facing up on top of your legs. The jaw is relaxed, and the tongue is pressed against the roof of the mouth just behind the top teeth. Inhale through the nose for 4 seconds, then hold for 4 seconds. Exhale through the nose for 4 seconds, then hold for 4 seconds. Repeat for up to six cycles. This should not be stressful, so adjust the time and number of cycles according to how you feel. As the 4-second cycle becomes easier, lengthen to 6, 8, and then 10 seconds.

4-4-6-2 Breathing

This exercise focuses on slowing the rate of respiration. The exhalation is longer than the inhalation to engage the parasympathetic nervous system, and the holds slow the rate of breathing. This breath practice is similar to box breathing, except the times are different. It should feel a little easier than a box-breathing session because the hold following the exhalation is not as long. This exercise reduces feelings of fear, anger, and impulsivity. Use this exercise any time of day and as often as needed before or during breaks in training or competition to relax and reduce anxiety or after competition or training to promote recovery.

To begin, sit upright on a chair with the feet flat on the floor or in a cross-legged position on the ground. Rest the arms at the sides with palms facing up on top of the legs. The jaw is relaxed, and the tongue is pressed against the roof of the mouth just behind the top teeth. Inhale through the nose for four seconds, and then hold for four seconds. Exhale through the nose for six seconds, and then hold for two seconds. Repeat for four to six cycles.

Pursed-Lips Breathing

The focus of this exercise is on the exhalation. Exhale through pursed lips to activate the abdominal muscles and make it easier to extend the exhalation. This technique helps keep the airways open so you can remove air quickly from the lungs. By pursing your lips on an exhalation, you are able to relieve shortness of breath and calm down. Use this exercise before training or competition to not only activate exhalation muscles but also to calm the nervous system. You can also use it during training or competition to recover or control emotions and after training or competition to recover. You can also use it before sleep.

To begin, sit in an upright position on a chair with the feet flat on the floor or sit in a cross-legged position on the ground. The arms are resting at your sides with palms facing up on top of the legs. The jaw is relaxed, and the tongue is pressed against the roof of the mouth just behind the top teeth. Inhale through the nose for 4 seconds, then take a brief pause. Purse the lips like you're blowing through a straw, and exhale through the mouth for 8 to 12 seconds. Repeat for up to five breaths when used during training or competing, and perform the exercise for three to five minutes after training or competition to recover.

Body Scanning

The objective of body scanning is to create full-body awareness in the present moment and to calm the mind and body. This can be helpful when you feel you have lost control of your emotions. Use this practice before or after training. You can also use this in the morning to start your day with a meditation practice.

Begin from one of these positions: Stand tall with a neutral spine, lie faceup on the ground, sit in a chair with the feet flat on the floor, or sit cross-legged on the ground. Blow all the air out of the lungs through the mouth, then take a normal inhalation through the nose, followed by a brief pause before you exhale normally through the nose. Perform five or six of these breaths to relax the body and create a slow breathing rate.

Once the body feels calm, focus your attention by imagining you're guiding a spotlight. First focus it between the eyebrows. Move the spotlight from the forehead to the entire front of the face. Then move it to the shoulders, chest, abdomen, hips, knees, ankles, and feet. Once you have scanned the front of the body, scan the back by working from the ankles up. Take as much time as you need to focus on specific parts of the body. Spend two to five seconds shining the spotlight on each body part while breathing slowly through the nose. Scan the body for 5 to 10 minutes.

Humming and Hissing

In this exercise you will choose whether to make a humming sound or hissing sound while exhaling. Humming and hissing are soothing sounds that promote calmness. This exercise produces nitric oxide that works as a vasodilator, engages the parasympathetic nervous system, and lowers the heart rate and blood pressure. Use this exercise in the morning upon waking to set the nervous system into a parasympathetic state and to produce nitric oxide. Use this exercise after training or competition to recover and shift the body to a parasympathetic state, or before bed to wind down. Perform this exercise for three to five minutes. It can be used daily.

To begin, sit upright on a chair with the feet flat on the floor or sit cross-legged on the ground. Rest the arms at the sides with your palms facing up on top of the legs. The jaw is relaxed, and the tongue is pressed against the roof of the mouth just behind the top teeth. Inhale through the nose for 4 seconds, then take a brief pause before exhaling through the nose for 8 to 12 seconds while making a humming or hissing sound, whichever you prefer. To hum, keep your lips gently sealed and feel a vibration in your throat. To hiss, use your tongue to create a slight resistance in the air as you gently exhale through the mouth. The lips are barely open as you exhale. You should feel calm while your mind focuses on either the hum or hiss.

Mindfulness Breathing

In this exercise you become mindful of your breathing by counting six continuous breaths and following them in your mind. Mindfulness breathing connects the mind with the body. By consciously slowing the breath, the limbic system and brainstem settle down with it and you are able to balance and control emotions. This opens space in your consciousness where you can become more aware of the moment. Use this exercise any time you feel anxious or stressed.

To begin, sit upright on a chair with the feet flat on the floor or sit cross-legged on the ground. Rest your arms at your sides with your palms facing up on top of your legs. The jaw is relaxed, and the tongue is pressed against the roof of the mouth just behind the top teeth. Inhale and exhale through the nose. Remain still as you become aware of your breath. You are not focused on a specific cadence or pauses in the breath. Simply pay attention to the natural rhythm of your breath. Count six breaths in your mind.

Alternate-Nostril Breathing

Alternate-nostril breathing is a popular mindfulness breathing technique. This exercise involves breathing cycles in which you inhale through one nostril while plugging the other one. Studies have shown that people who performed alternate-nostril breathing were able to reduce their stress levels and improve their heart rate and heart rate variability, breathing rate, and overall cardiovascular health (Sharma et al. 2013). This exercise can be used daily before or after training or competition. This breathing practice is meditative and relaxing, which makes mornings or evenings a great time to use it. It helps clear mental space and create a balanced nervous system.

To begin, sit upright on a chair with the feet flat on the floor or sit cross-legged on the ground. Place your left hand on your left knee. The jaw is relaxed, and the tongue is pressed against the roof of the mouth just behind the top teeth. Exhale completely through the mouth, and with your right hand, place your thumb over your right nostril (see figure *a*). Inhale through your left nostril, then close the left nostril with your index finger (see figure *b*). Open the right nostril by lifting your thumb as you exhale through the right nostril (see figure *c*). After you have exhaled through the right nostril, inhale through the right nostril, close it with the thumb (see figure *d*), open the left nostril by lifting your index finger, then exhale through the left nostril (see figure *e*). This completes one cycle. The cycle always finishes with an exhalation through the left nostril. This will finish the breathing cycle in a parasympathetic state. When you inhale and exhale through the left nostril, the body cools itself and relaxes. Inhaling and exhaling through the right nostril turns up the heat in the body and gives you energy. Repeat the cycle for 5 to 10 minutes.

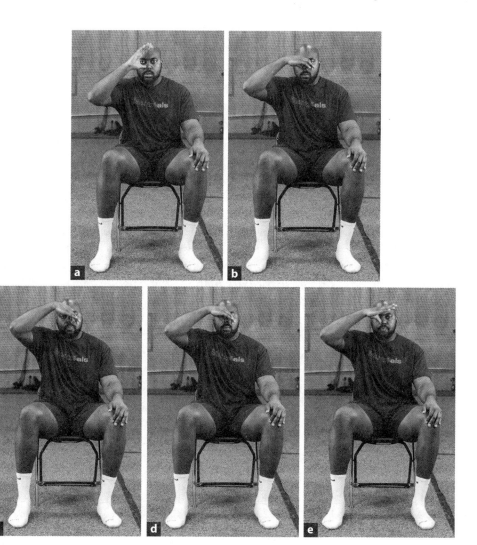

Ujjayi Breathing

Ujjayi breathing is commonly translated as "victorious breath" and has been used for thousands of years to enhance the hatha yoga practice. This exercise improves concentration while releasing tension from the body and regulates heating to warm the body. Use this exercise to warm up for training or competition. You can also use this breathing practice while sitting in a cold tub, which will be further explored in the next chapter.

To begin, sit upright on a chair with the feet flat on the floor or sit cross-legged on the ground. Rest your arms and place your hands on your knees with palms facing up. The jaw is relaxed, and the tongue is pressed against the roof of the mouth just behind the top teeth. Seal your lips and breathe in and out through your nose. Inhale through the nose slower and deeper than normal while feeling like the air is being restricted in the back of the throat. Then exhale while making sure to constrict the muscles in the back of the throat. This will create a noise, and some people consider this style of breathing to sound like Darth Vader from *Star Wars*. The outflow typically happens faster than the inflow of this breathing practice. For beginners, take a normal inhalation and exhalation while constricting the throat. If you are able to consistently perform the exhalation, create the same resistance and sound on the inhalation.

If you're having trouble making the sound, try inhaling deeper than normal, and when you exhale, open your mouth wide and make the sound "haaah." This should be similar to the sound made when fogging up the mirror. When you can make the sound while exhaling through the mouth, practice with the lips sealed. Perform this exercise for 5 to 10 minutes.

Double Inhalation With Extended Exhale

In this exercise you will take two inhalations through the nose and exhale through the mouth. Use this exercise when you are stressed or anxious. It immediately induces a sense of calm in just a few breaths.

To begin, sit upright with feet flat on the floor or cross-legged on the ground. Rest your arms at your sides with palms facing up on the legs. The jaw is relaxed, and the tongue is pressed against the roof of the mouth just behind the top teeth. Through the nose, take a deep inhalation into the belly followed by a brief pause. Take another nasal inhalation into the chest. This should feel like a sip of air. Exhale through the mouth for double the length of the inhalation. Repeat for one to three cycles.

Straw Breathing

In this exercise you will exhale through a drinking straw after inhaling through the nose. This exercise increases the length of the exhalation, calms the body, and promotes a parasympathetic state. You can perform this exercise twice a day: in the morning and evening.

To begin, sit upright either on a chair with the feet flat on the floor or cross-legged on the ground. Rest your arms at your sides. The jaw is relaxed, and the tongue is pressed against the roof of the mouth just behind the top teeth. Keep one hand on the same-side knee and the straw in the other. Exhale all the air through your mouth before taking a natural inhalation through the nose (see figure *a*). Once you have inhaled, place the straw in your mouth. You can either gently hold it to your lips with your thumb and index finger or keep the straw in your mouth without holding it and place your hand on the same-side knee. After inhaling through the nose, exhale fully through the drinking straw (see figure *b*). Repeat for five minutes.

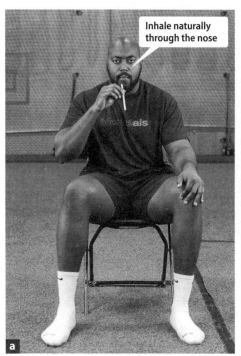
Inhale naturally through the nose

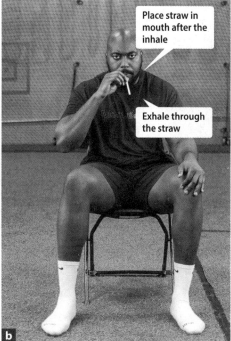
Place straw in mouth after the inhale

Exhale through the straw

Sitali Breath

This breathing exercise is different from most of the practices in this chapter. You will inhale through the mouth through a curled tongue and exhale through the nose. This is also known as "cooling breath." Use this exercise in training or competition during moments of stress.

To begin, sit upright either on a chair with the feet flat on the floor or cross-legged on the ground. Rest your arms at your sides with the palms facing up on top of the legs. The jaw is relaxed. Close your eyes, and curl the edges of your tongue together. Inhale through an open mouth (see figure *a*). Breathe in slower and deeper than normal. Then close your mouth and exhale through your nose until you run out of air (see figure *b*). This should be slow and quiet and shouldn't be stressful. Repeat for three to six breaths. If you cannot curl your tongue, perform the exercise by resting your tongue on the top of your bottom teeth. You will still inhale through the mouth with a relaxed jaw. Close the mouth and exhale through the nose.

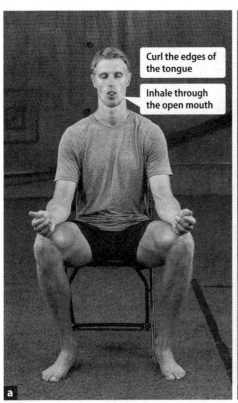

Curl the edges of the tongue

Inhale through the open mouth

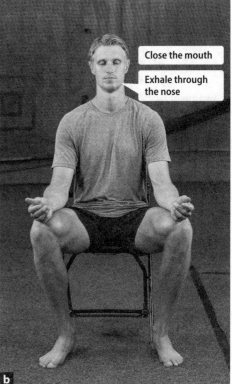

Close the mouth

Exhale through the nose

Body Hug Deep Breathing

This exercise triggers the vagus nerve and promotes full diaphragmatic breathing that allows 360-degree expansion of the rib cage. It also engages the parasympathetic nervous system. This exercise can be done before training or competition. And it is beneficial to use it to start your day so you can become mindful of your body and breath. A single breath helps center the mind and body for the day.

To begin, stand tall or lie faceup on the ground. Wrap your right arm around your body, resting the hand under the armpit. Wrap the left arm around the abdomen below the right arm. Be careful of your hand position because digging your fingers into your body can trigger the sympathetic nervous system. Keep your hands open to allow your breath to push your torso against the palms and base of the fingers. While hugging your body at these angles, you should feel a full inhalation into both hands as you breathe horizontally and fill the body (see figure *a*). You should feel the body go back in as you exhale (see figure *b*). Inhale deeply through the nose for six seconds, hold for six seconds, exhale through the nose for eight seconds, and then take a brief pause. Repeat for six breaths.

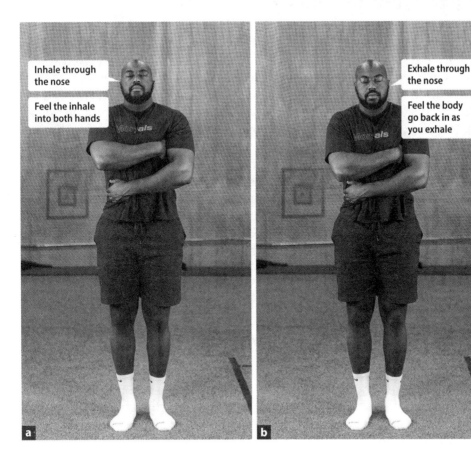

Wim Hof Breathing

Wim Hof, an extreme athlete also known as the Iceman, is known for his world records for cold and underwater swims and for climbing mountains shirtless. (See the sidebar in chapter 3 on page 46.) His adventures and feats have helped researchers better understand physiology and how the body and mind respond to stress.

The Wim Hof method involves a deep inhalation, followed by relaxed exhalations, and prolonged breath holds to control the body and mind through the breath. This training is related to tummo meditation, an ancient technique practiced by monks in Tibetan Buddhism. The benefits of the Wim Hof method include improved clarity and concentration, stress reduction, and better sleep and energy. While the Wim Hof method is commonly used in conjunction with cold exposure, this is not necessary to reap the emotion-regulating benefits. Here we'll explore the breathing protocols and their benefits. The following are modified breathing practices based on the Wim Hof method.

Beginner Wim Hof Method

Use this practice to become familiar with the Wim Hof method. Find a quiet space and lie on your back with a pillow under your head; this will properly position the neck and spine. Relax the shoulders and chest. Your arms are relaxed at your sides, knees are bent, and feet are flat on the floor.

Take 30 deep breaths as fast as you can while focusing on bringing the air deep into your belly. Bring the air in through the nose and let it out through pursed lips. Imagine your body is a wave as you breathe in and breathe out, filling up the belly with air as the wave rises. The wave subsides as the belly empties on the exhalation. At the end of 30 breaths, exhale the last breath, leaving a quarter of the air in the lungs. Hold this breath for as long as possible. Once you feel a strong urge to breathe, take a massive inhalation and hold it for another 15 seconds. Ideally, this inhalation is through the nose, but if you need to breathe through the mouth, that's OK. Exhale after the 15-second hold. Repeat this pattern for three sets, adding a fourth as you become stronger.

As you begin, don't worry about how long you hold your breath. Instead, pay attention to the feelings and space created through the practice. After the intense breathing you should feel a sense of calmness and alertness. If during the practice you feel lightheadedness, tingling, or like you will pass out, stop the practice and resume slow nasal breathing until the symptoms subside.

During this practice notice the sound of your breath. Loud and fast breathing sounds signal an intense breathing practice. Quieter breathing is naturally slower. If you want to push aggressively and create a sympathetic response, then breathe loudly during inhalation. If you're looking for a parasympathetic response, breathe in deeply through the nose and out through the mouth quietly. This will naturally slow your breathing.

Elevated Wim Hof Method

This elevated version of the Wim Hof method uses a double inhalation. You will take two inhalations for every exhalation. This double inhalation creates a better exchange of oxygen and carbon dioxide in the alveoli. Breathing deeply into the lungs and then extending the exhalation promotes a parasympathetic response.

Find a quiet space and lie on your back with a pillow under your head. This positions the neck and spine properly. Relax the shoulders and chest. The arms are relaxed at your sides, your knees are bent, and your feet are flat on the floor.

Inhale through the nose and into the belly. Focus on reaching 90 percent of your inhalation capacity on this first movement. Take the next 10 percent of the inhalation into the chest, still through the nose. At maximum inhalation, fully exhale the air through the mouth. Pause briefly after the exhalation, then take another inhalation with 90 percent of the air into the belly followed by 10 percent into the chest. Feel as though you're creating a wave in your body as you feel the air coming in and going out. This breathing practice is continuous, without stops, pauses, or breath holds.

Continue this practice as follows: 5 to 10 minutes for beginners, 15 to 30 minutes for intermediate level, and 45 to 75 minutes for advanced level. This practice is best for a recovery day. Pair this with a sauna and cold tub or a walk in nature. You can use it before training or competition to spark adrenaline and focus, but only for 3 to 5 minutes. Extending this practice past that can tax the body and use energy that is better reserved for performance (MacCormick 2020).

Holotropic Breathing

Holotropic breathing is used for emotional healing and has been said to alter an individual's state of consciousness. Typically, this fast-paced breathing is undertaken with a guide who supports the healing process, and it is essential that it be paired with music. Consult with a doctor or medical professional before entering a holotropic breathing session.

Research has shown that holotropic breathing can improve one's self-awareness (Miller and Nielsen 2015). Some have used this practice to not only enhance their perspective on life but also to build self-esteem and eliminate negative thinking. This practice has helped people overcome trauma and tragic experiences, allowing them to find purpose and live life with intention. This unconventional practice was developed in the 1970s by psychiatrist Stanislav Grof and his wife, Christina Grof, who was a psychotherapist, to achieve altered states of consciousness (without using drugs) as a potential therapeutic tool. As a spiritual practice, it is trademarked through the Grof Holotropic Foundation.

During holotropic breathing practice, the individual uses controlled fast-paced breathing to hyperventilate and deprive themselves of oxygen. Prolonged breathing practice with limited oxygen is said to create an altered state of consciousness. These practices can be prolonged for hours and be done in a one-on-one or group setting. Most practitioners suggest supporting the breath practice by following it with a creative act. That could be journaling, painting, drawing, or group discussion.

If you are interested in holotropic breathing, seek an experienced guide. This practice takes place outside of the athletic platform and is not for everyone. As a therapeutic experience, holotropic breathing is meant to help people break through the avoidance barriers in their life. It has been shown to decrease stress and chronic pain, alleviate depression, and decrease the negative effects of previous trauma. Use this practice of self-exploration away from training and performing. It is not meant to improve athletic performance or stimulate a ready state for training or competition. It is an emotional healing process that can help you overcome the negativity bias and barriers standing in your way.

Balance Breathing

The exercises presented here use balance techniques to add an extra stimulus to your breathing patterns and can be used before training or competition. The main goal of balance techniques paired with breathing is to help your body control itself during a challenge. Improving your balance also aids in injury prevention, improved cognition, muscle coordination, and mindful breathing. Perform balance exercises up to three times a day. Here are a few key points before you begin these exercises:

- Each of the exercises is meant to take place as a standalone practice, and you determine how often and how long you want to practice each exercise.
- Perform the exercises barefoot so you can use the big toe to create stability.
- Use nasal breathing when performing these exercises.
- If you find you are holding your breath, relax the body and remind yourself to keep breathing.

Balance Breathing Warm-Up

Before you begin the balance breathing exercises, warm up your feet. This warm-up will also help build toe and foot strength. Do this warm-up every time you perform one of the exercises that follow.

1. Stand tall with the feet shoulder-width apart and pointing forward. Arms are loose and free, resting at your sides with the hands open. While balancing, use your arms to help maintain balance if you need to.

2. Take normal breaths in and out through the nose, and continue nasal breathing throughout.

3. Starting with the right foot, hold four toes down while lifting the big toe off the ground (see figure *a*). Hold for 10 seconds.

4. Push the big toe down while lifting the other four toes off the ground (see figure *b*). Hold for 10 seconds.

5. Hold the big toe and pinkie toe on the ground while lifting the three middle toes (see figure *c*). Hold for 10 seconds.

6. Lift the right foot off the ground and perform 10 circles clockwise and 10 circles counterclockwise while moving from the ankle and pointing the big toe forward (see figure *d*).

7. Repeat steps 3 through 6 on the left foot. You only need to do this once through on each foot.

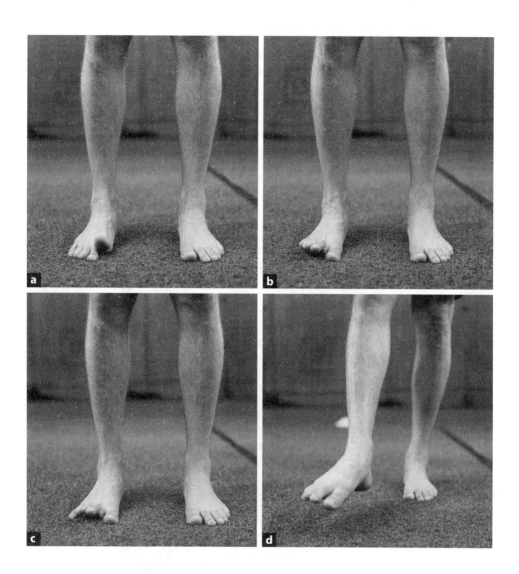

Stand on One Foot on Flat Surface

This exercise builds ankle and foot strength while coordinating your breath with the stillness of the exercise. Practice this before or after training and competition to create mindfulness and awareness of the breath.

1. Stand tall with the feet shoulder-width apart and pointing forward. Your arms are at your sides, and the palms are facing out in front of you.
2. Lift the left foot and balance on the right foot (see figure).
3. Hold this position while taking six normal inhalations and exhalations through the nose. There is no specific breathing protocol. Breathe at a consistent cadence with a brief pause after the inhalation and exhalation.
4. Repeat up to three times on each leg.

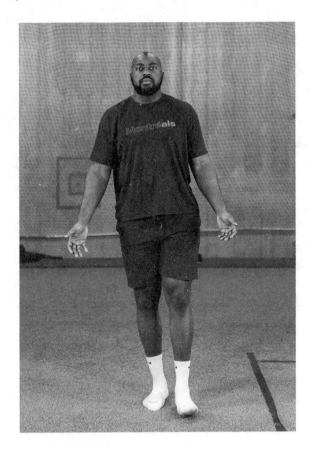

Flamingo Stand on Flat Surface

This exercise builds ankle and foot strength while coordinating the rib cage with your hips, keeping the spine neutral, and expanding the rib cage 360 degrees while balancing on one leg. Practice this before or after training and competition to create mindfulness and awareness of the breath.

1. Stand tall with the feet shoulder-width apart and pointing forward. The hands are near your sides, palms facing out.

2. Inhale through the nose and lift the left leg by bringing the knee up to hip height and keeping the hip at a 90-degree angle (see figure). Take a normal inhalation followed by a normal exhalation. Keep the rib cage over the hips and the spine neutral while balancing on one foot.

3. Hold the position while nasal breathing for 15 seconds.

4. Repeat on the other leg.

5. Repeat one to three times on each leg.

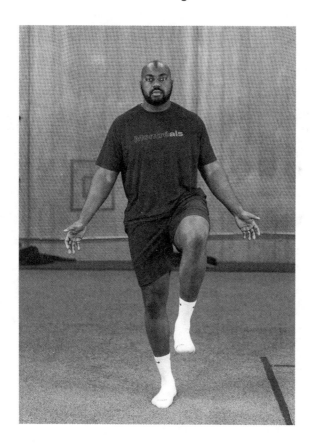

Heel-to-Toe Walk on Flat Surface

The goal of this exercise is to maintain balance while coordinating your breath with the movement. The next exercise, Paced Breathing While Walking, will extend this exercise. To perform this exercise, follow these steps:

1. Mark a 20-foot (6 meters) line on the ground.
2. At one end, stand tall with the feet shoulder-width apart and pointing forward. Hold the arms out at shoulder level so they are parallel with the floor.
3. Walk forward along the line, placing the heel of one foot in front of the other foot's toes as you move forward (see figures *a-b*).
4. Inhale through the nose on the first step, then exhale through the nose on the next step. Continue this pattern as you move forward.
5. When you reach the end of the line, walk backward in the same manner, with the toes to the heel of the other foot, and continue the same breathing pattern.
6. Repeat one to five times.

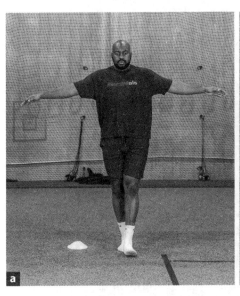 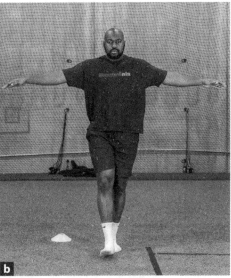

Grounding Practices

Electricity is everywhere. Electricity is even required for our nervous system to send signals to our brain and body about the experience it is perceiving from the outside world. This helps explain the benefits of grounding our bare feet to the earth's surface. Grounding has been shown to improve our health through the transfer of energy from the ground into our body. The connection the body has with the earth has shown to improve heart rate variability, oxygen consumption, and shifting from a sympathetic state to a parasympathetic state. This helps create mental space for our conscious mind to think rational and feel calmer, eliminating limbic brain activity.

Spend 20 to 40 minutes walking barefoot through a safe, grassy area while nasal breathing only. Focus on each step with your eyes. This will keep the breathing rate slow while also keeping your feet from stepping where they shouldn't. Perform this three to five times a week. You can use grounding right away in the morning to promote an early parasympathetic state and slow breathing. This will help stabilize your energy for the day. Any time you are grounded, parasympathetic activity takes over, which naturally slows breathing. Spending time with your bare feet on the ground will help bring awareness to slow, rhythmic breathing.

Paced Breathing While Walking

The objective of this exercise is to walk while counting. This trains the timing of your movement with your breath. If you are performing a 1:1 ratio, you are most likely walking faster than during a 4:4 ratio. The first number is how many steps you take while you inhale, and the second number is how many steps you take while you exhale. You are forcing cognitive awareness through movement and being mindful of the breath. Mental and physical focus are required to maintain the sequences.

Beginner to Intermediate

Start with a 1:1 ratio and walk slowly as you synchronize your breath with the movement. It shouldn't take long to get the rhythm down. As you feel comfortable, increase the ratio to 2:2 and eventually to 4:4. If you have been exposed to this training before, start at the 3:3 ratio.

- *1:1*—Step down with one foot and inhale, then step down with the other and exhale.
- *2:2*—Take two steps while you inhale, then take two steps while you exhale.
- *3:3*—Take three steps while you inhale, then take three steps while you exhale.
- *4:4*—Take four steps while you inhale, then take four steps while you exhale.

Advanced

Once you are proficient in the beginner to intermediate protocols, move ahead to the advanced protocols.

Triangle Sequence

The triangle sequence is similar to the beginner and intermediate protocols, except you will inhale for a specific number of steps, then hold your breath for a specific number of steps, and finally exhale for a specific number of steps. Perform these protocols in order.

1. Four steps inhale, five steps hold, five steps exhale (5 to 10 minutes total)
2. Three steps inhale, four steps hold, three steps exhale (5 to 10 minutes total)
3. Two steps inhale, three steps hold, two steps exhale (5 to 10 minutes total)
4. Four steps inhale, four steps hold, two steps exhale (5 to 10 minutes total)

Custom Sequence

There is no hold in this sequence. As you improve, you can develop longer steps or fewer steps to challenge the sequence on both the inhalation and exhalation.

1. One step inhale, three steps exhale (5 to 10 minutes total)
2. Four steps inhale, one step exhale (5 to 10 minutes total)

In addition to the advanced protocols, you can further challenge your concentration by placing obstacles in the drill. Walk in a straight line 20 to 50 yards (18-46 meters) back and forth for the time allocated to the exercise. Next, place boxes, hurdles, cones, or balance beams in the path that you must walk on, over, or around to complete the distance. Place a stick or other obstacles that you must duck under or jump over. Keep the breathing consistent regardless of the obstacles. You will naturally begin to step more quickly on the higher breath counts, but try to stay relaxed, even, and calm.

Through this chapter, you have learned many styles of recovery. No single protocol is perfect or appropriate for everyone. Try them all to find the one that provides you the best recovery. The goal is to slow the breathing rate and start the process of adaptation. The beginning of the chapter touched on how to slow the breath and the concept of EPOC breathing. The remainder of the chapter outlined many breathing practices to use in the moment of training or competition. When you have just a few minutes to recover, you want to rely on the protocol you know works for you. After training or competition, it is optimal to spend 10 to 30 minutes slowing and controlling your breath to recover. Practices such as the Wim Hof method or holotropic breathing are best used outside of the performance arena. Try these practices on off days and experiment with environmental stressors and journaling. Use the balance exercises and paced breathing with walking exercises on off days or lighter training days. Chapter 9 will cover environmental stress and ways to train your breathing while being immersed into cold or hot temperatures.

Environmental Stress Exercises

An athlete's ability to embrace stress and learn from it to enhance performance is a powerful tool. This chapter teaches you how to control your breathing while deliberately placing yourself in situations made stressful by cold or heat. Research into mindset shows that when someone deliberately does something they believe will be good for them, it results in different physiological effects than if something were happening to them that they had no control over. A study of Navy SEALs found that a stress-is-enhancing mindset outperforms a stress-is-debilitating mindset (Smith, Young, and Crum 2020). In this chapter, we explore cold and heat training and protocols so you can add this impactful way of training to your repertoire.

Our natural survival instinct is to seek comfort in temperatures that keep us around 68 to 72 degrees Fahrenheit (20-22.2 °C). By getting outside of this comfort zone and stressing the cellular functioning of the body either by using heat and cold in the same session or focusing on one temperature extreme, we strengthen our physiological systems. We lower our daily respiratory rate, improve our muscle tissue, and raise our threshold for handling stress. Evidence shows that we are at our best—physically harder, mentally tougher, and spiritually sounder—after experiencing the same discomforts our early ancestors were exposed to every day (Easter 2021). The lack of temperature change caused by indoor lifestyles and misalignment with nature has taken us far from our ancestorial upbringing, and it continues to weaken the nervous system. By intentionally placing ourselves into the heat or cold, we become our best physically, mentally, and even spiritually.

Cold Exposure

Cold exposure to improve athletic performance has drawn a lot of interest in recent years. The athletic feats and training method of Wim Hof, known as the Iceman (see page 46), are gaining worldwide attention. Using cold exposure to train mentally and physically is a powerful tool that deepens your relationship with the physiological sensations that come with the experience and produces higher cognition, emotional control, and improved endurance.

What Is Cold Exposure?

Controlled exposure to cold that causes stress creates healthy and positive adaptations that improve mental, emotional, and physical health. You can put your body in a cold state in many ways. It can be as simple as taking a cold shower, standing outside in the winter, or lying in snow. It can also go as far as full-body immersion into ice tubs, bathtubs, lakes, creeks, or anything that allows a full-body soak into temperatures below 60 degrees Fahrenheit (15.5 °C). By learning how to use the breath in these controlled cold environments, you will be able to lower your respiration rate and quiet the reptilian, or limbic, brain activity that takes place in stressful situations.

Cold exposure is another way of saying cold thermogenesis, and is the process in which the body creates its own heat while exposed to temperatures far below optimal conditions. Think of a time you were cold and you started to shiver, your skin became tight, the hairs on the body stood up, and parts of your body turned red. This was caused by a type of thermogenesis. Members of the cold-exposure communities around the world call this the body's heat vent. A heat vent is formed as a response to cold entering the body.

When the body's heat vent is activated, the cold activates brown adipose tissue (BAT), or brown fat. Most of the body's fat is white fat, which stores extra energy, and too much accumulated in the body leads to obesity. Brown fat breaks down blood sugar (glucose) and fat molecules to create heat and help the body maintain body temperature. This thermogenic fat can increase core body temperature, and acting as the body's furnace, it can increase core metabolism. Thermogenic fat, or brown fat, helps the body stay lean and reduces general inflammation.

The ease with which we can avoid cold temperature through apparel, artificial temperature control, and lack of outside exposure negatively affects the stimulation of BAT. The more we get away from nature, the less we use the body's existing systems to produce energy and maintain homeostasis. This leaves us with bodies insulated by white fat around the organs, and this weighs heavy on our breathing muscles, forcing more work during respiration, especially inhalation, which is an active movement. With additional weight and a restricted rib cage, we have to work harder to expand the surface area of the lungs through inhalation. This could be the reason for a rise in respiration rate as people become obese.

The more exposure to the cold, the higher the levels of beneficial brown fat. Therefore, cold exposure should be on your daily to-do list and eventually become a habitual act that builds healthy breathing and mindful moments into your daily life.

How Does Cold Exposure Work?

When you're exposed to cold temperatures, your body has to work harder to stay at homeostasis and regulate core temperature. In addition, hormones such as epinephrine and norepinephrine are activated when your body is exposed to cold. Both of these hormones—which are behind the fight-or-flight response—help activate heart and blood activity through the adrenaline produced because of the exposure to cold. While cold is a stressor, it's a positive stress. Similar to being exposed to morning sunlight, when you are exposed to cold you produce cortisol, which is a stress hormone but one that promotes energy and healthy metabolism throughout the day.

Cold exposure stresses the body, in particular the nervous system. Just as you train in the weight room or run sprints to improve performance, you want to put the body through stress to learn how to adapt and become a better functioning athlete. In addition to the external signs of cold exposure (shivering, tight skin, red skin, erect body hair), inside the body the blood vessels constrict, which increases the respiration rate. This is the acute stress response you experience when first exposed to the cold. Over repeated exposure, you adapt and raise your resilience level, which minimizes your body's fight-or-flight response. Controlled exposure to a stressor results in adaptation to that stressor.

What Are the Benefits of Cold Exposure?

Cold exposure can be used to improve both mental performance and physical performance. As you explore the experience of cold exposure, it helps to know the benefits that come with it.

- Speeds metabolism
- Improves brown adipose tissue, which helps burn white fat
- Reduces general inflammation
- Improves quality of sleep
- Improves immune response
- Increases energy levels and focus
- Creates resiliency and strengthens the mind
- Relieves symptoms caused by autoimmune disease
- Releases norepinephrine and adrenaline in the body
- Increases cell longevity and tissue health

What Are the Safety Concerns for Cold Exposure?

If cold exposure is overused or used at the wrong time, the body stays in a fight-or-flight state, burning energy and leading to severe fatigue. Worse, the cold can cause hypothermia or frostbite, which are dangerous. It is unlikely that the protocols in this chapter will lead to hypothermia or severe fatigue; however, it is important to be aware of the potential.

Watch for signs and symptoms such as dehydration, numbness, intense shivering, memory loss, disorientation, slurred speech, and extreme exhaustion. These are early warning signs of danger, and you should remove yourself from the cold immediately. If the cold is overwhelming, the natural reaction is to hyperventilate and breathe into the upper chest through your mouth. You want to maintain calm nasal breathing during cold exposure to keep calm and maintain mental clarity. If the breath becomes stressed, so does the body.

Cold Exposure Exercises

In earlier chapters, we discussed extreme athlete Wim Hof and his athletic accomplishments and training method that combines breathing practice with cold exposure. The exercises here use breathing protocols similar to those that Wim Hof uses to build tolerance to stress and pair that with cold. Breath work paired with cold exposure is an effective modality for training to control your physiological and psychological responses to a stressful stimulus. As this skill improves, you will be able to perform in longer flow states while lengthening the mental space between stimulus and response. This increases your resiliency not only in performance but in life as well. Remember, you don't need to stay in the cold very long, just long enough to get your breathing under control. That is all it takes to begin the process of adaptation.

The exercises in this section explore different levels of cold immersion. The goal is to find the level that works for you that is safe but also causes you to be uncomfortable. Note that if you can't control your breathing during cold exposure or cold immersion, you are not adapting. Use cold-immersion protocols in the mornings within two hours of waking or at least four hours after training or competition. Cold immersion should be avoided or used minimally in the evenings because of the potential for sleep interruption and should not be used immediately before bed (this will be discussed in more detail later).

Beginner Cold Immersion: Cold Exposure

These beginner cold-immersion practices are the easiest and best way to control the stress response. They are used to control breathing and to learn how you handle stress. You can expose the face, hand, and feet to cold to build endurance and prepare for eventual full-body immersion.

Face in Cold Water

This practice uses cold water on the face by either splashing or submerging in a controlled environment such as a shower, outdoor hose, sink, or bucket of cold water. Expose your face to cold water for 15 to 60 seconds. You can expose your face to cold water daily in the mornings or even several times throughout the day.

Splashing Cold Water on the Face

Splash cold water on your face during breaks in training or competition to activate a parasympathetic response, which lowers the respiration and heart rate. The impact of vagus nerve stimulation on the nervous system can also help bring you back into the moment and back into a mindful state.

Pour cold water into your hands and splash the water around the eyes and just below them. Keep your eyes closed and maintain nasal breathing throughout. Before splashing the water on the face, hold your breath. It should be instinctive to hold your breath while splashing water on your face, but maintain awareness and be mindful of a short breath hold. Following the hold, continue nasal breathing. Splash the water for 10 to 15 seconds.

Full-Face Submersion

For this technique, hold your breath while placing your entire face in cold water. This will stimulate the vagus nerve and elicit a parasympathetic response, lowering the respiration and heart rate. Use this technique following a sauna session or intense training session or before or after a breathing practice to start the adaptation from a sympathetic to parasympathetic state.

Breathe normally through the nose, then hold your breath on either the inhalation or exhalation and submerge your face underwater for 15 to 20 seconds. The breath hold will be easier on the inhalation because the lungs have a reserve volume. When you come up, continue to breathe normally through the nose.

Hands and Feet in Cold Water

This cold-water immersion practice consists of submerging the hands or feet into cold water for a specific amount of time. The initial response to cold on the hands and feet is a strong vasoconstriction, leading to a rapid decrease in hand and feet temperature, which impairs tactile sensitivity, dexterity, and muscle contractile characteristics while increasing pain and sympathetic activity. This also decreases motor function and performance (Cheung 2015). These techniques help strengthen and build resilience in the extremities. Use these techniques on off days or at least two hours before or after training.

Place both hands in a bowl of ice water large enough to submerge the hands, or place both feet in a bucket of ice water so that the feet are fully submerged to just above the ankles. Begin by inhaling through the nose for four seconds, hold for two seconds, then exhale through the nose or mouth for seven seconds. Continue this breathing pattern throughout the exercise. For beginners, hold the hands underwater for two minutes (8-10 breaths) to four minutes (16-20 breaths). Once you feel you have met the adaptation needed while controlling the breath, increase to six minutes (24-30 breaths) to eight minutes (32-40 breaths). Do not exceed eight minutes. Water temperature and submersion times will depend on how long you can tolerate the stress. If you cannot stay submerged for the time you're aiming for, increase the temperature of the water or shorten the time.

Cold Shower

A cold shower is one of the most popular and most efficient ways to achieve full-body exposure to the cold (although it's not as effective as full-body cold-water immersion, which is discussed later). A cold shower reduces inflammatory cytokine levels, activates brown adipose tissue to burn fat, and induces a hormone response, which all strengthen the immune system. The cold shower releases adrenaline, which helps maintain energy throughout the day. The cold shower can serve you well during travel or long delays in competition, and it dilates the blood vessels and helps release nitric oxide. This is important for the flow of oxygen into the muscle tissue. The slight increase in glucose and oxygen uptake in the organs and muscles can help you reduce symptoms of jet lag and decrease fatigue during strenuous training or competition.

There is no specific breathing protocol for the cold-shower techniques. Beginners may feel as though it's difficult to control their breathing and could begin to hyperventilate. In this case the goal is to first slow the breathing and then control the breath while breathing only through the mouth. After each inhalation, take a two- to four-second hold and lengthen the exhalation. The length of the exhalation should be double the length of the inhalation. If you don't find it difficult to breathe in a cold shower, focus on nasal breathing only while being mindful of the cold touching the entire body. After a cold shower you will notice a sense of clarity and energy that will be sustained throughout the day.

Hot-to-Cold Shower

The hot-to-cold shower is a common way to practice cold exposure. Contrast therapy, in which you alternate the temperature of the water, can be therapeutic and relaxing. Using hot water also minimizes the stress of a strictly cold shower. Taking a hot-to-cold shower before going out in the cold eases the transition into the cold and lessens the shock of the cold environment.

Take a normal hot or warm shower. Once you have finished showering, turn on the cold water and let it hit the front of your body (face, chest, legs) for 15 seconds. Turn around and let the water hit the back of your body (head, back, legs) for 15 seconds, and finish by having the cold water hit your face again for a few seconds. Allow the water to hit the entire body and take your time in the shower to breathe and feel the impact of cold on all the body parts. You can take a hot-to-cold shower daily because finishing with 30 seconds of cold exposure will not affect the nervous system in a way that could affect training or competition. After the shower, dry off and warm up naturally. There is no need to seek a warming source. The body will warm itself quickly.

Cold-Only Shower

You can use a cold-only shower every morning to create alertness, focus, and energy for the day. This will trigger sympathetic activity for the duration of the shower, and the body will naturally shift into a parasympathetic state after the shower. Step into a cold shower and allow the water to hit the entire body, and expose the front and back for equal amounts of time. Try for two to five minutes while feeling the impact of cold on the body and being mindful of your breath. After the shower, dry off and warm up naturally. There is no need to seek a warming source. The body will warm itself quickly.

A cold-only shower can also be used every evening to create an initial shock to stimulate the sympathetic nervous system. This takes just 15 to 45 seconds in a cold shower. As the body warms naturally, it will fall into a parasympathetic state, allowing you to relax with a positive body temperature. Staying in the cold shower longer than 45 seconds will activate the body's heat vent, leading to higher body temperature as you head to bed, which could cause sleep disruptions.

Contrast Shower

A contrast shower can be used for relaxation, to promote a parasympathetic state, and for regeneration on recovery days. For this technique, take either a 5-minute or 10-minute shower that alternates between hot and cold as follows:

- Take a 5-minute shower, alternating between 20 seconds of cold water and 10 seconds of hot water. This will create 10 cycles of cold-to-hot contrasting. How you start is not as important as how you end—always finish on cold.

- Take a 10-minute shower in which you alternate between 30 seconds of cold water and 30 seconds of hot water. This will create 10 cycles of cold-to-hot contrasting, in which you spend equal amounts of time in the hot and the cold. Again, how you start is not as important as how you end—always finish on cold.

Moderate Cold Immersion: Full-Body Cold Exposure

Cold immersion takes place by submerging the entire body into a cold-water tub (see figure). This is considered a moderate level because this deliberate exposure to cold is used after experiencing the beginner exposures such as a cold shower or exposing the face, hands, or feet to the cold. The protocols in this section are the most common full-body cold-water immersion techniques. Keeping only the head above water, you will focus on the breath while the body undergoes stress beneath the water.

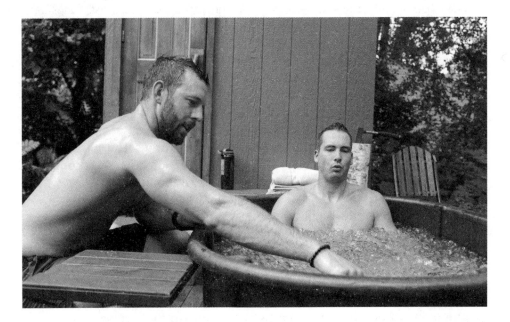

You will need a tub large enough to submerge your entire body up to the neck. Typically, a 100- to 150-gallon (378-568 liter) tub will fit your entire body without too much water spilling or splashing out. Stock tanks used for livestock can be found online or at local hardware stores. A bathtub works, too.

The length of the immersion and the temperature of the water depends on how you respond, feel, or anticipate entering the cold, which is unique to each person. How cold the water should be depends on your cold tolerance and metabolism, which you won't know beforehand. In general, the water should be cold enough that your reaction is "Whoa, I'd like to get out of this experience, but I can stay in safely." With this in mind, athletes are capable of controlling their breath immersed in water that is 35 degrees Fahrenheit (1.7 °C), but most athletic cold tubs are 50 to 60 degrees Fahrenheit (10-15.5 °C). This temperature allows for the adaptations needed to advance an athlete's performance, but dropping the temperature into the 30s (0.5-4 °C) introduces a deeper psychological component that helps strengthen the mind. The experience should be difficult but never feel unsafe. Here are general time guidelines for different temperatures:

50-59 Degrees Fahrenheit (10-15 °C)

- *Beginner*: 3 to 5 minutes
- *Intermediate*: 7 to 10 minutes
- *Advanced*: 15 to 20 minutes

40-49 Degrees Fahrenheit (4.4-9.4 °C)

- *Beginner*: 30 seconds to 1 minute
- *Intermediate*: 2 to 4 minutes
- *Advanced*: 4 to 7 minutes

33-39 Degrees Fahrenheit (0.5-3.9 °C)

- *Beginner*: Advised not to use
- *Intermediate*: 1 to 2 minutes
- *Advanced*: 2 to 5 minutes

By consistently exposing yourself to the cold, you will learn how to regulate your breathing and how to relax the body so you are in control while experiencing the shock and stress that comes with cold exposure. Use the following guidelines as you begin full-body immersion. Over time, you will discover the system that works best for you.

- If you are a beginner, you may want to start by submerging to just below the nipples. As you progress and feel comfortable, you can sit back in the tub and allow the water to rise above the chest to right around the collarbone.

- You do not need a specific breathing protocol before entering the tub. However, 10 minutes of ujjayi breathing (see page 158) or three rounds of Wim Hof breathing (see page 162) may help create heat in the body and focus.

- The goal during the full-body immersion is to keep the breath under control. The best breathing protocol is a four-second inhalation, a two-second hold, then a seven-second exhalation. Depending on your tolerance to cold, use one of the following gears to maintain this breathing protocol:
  - *High gear (low tolerance to cold)*: Mouth inhalation, mouth exhalation
  - *Middle gear (moderate tolerance to cold)*: Nasal inhalation, mouth exhalation
  - *Low gear (high tolerance to cold)*: Nasal inhalation, nasal exhalation

- Keep the arms crossed and place both hands in the armpits or bring your knees in close to the body while placing both hands in the armpits. This helps keep body heat in and also helps you maintain focus on your breath while your body feels safer in the cold.
- During the full-body immersion session, breathe horizontally and use the diaphragm to expand the rib cage. Avoid using auxiliary breathing muscles, evident by breathing into the neck or shoulders. The water pressure in the tub should create a force around the rib cage, which aids in proper breathing mechanics. This is another benefit of full-body immersion. In the shower, there is no water pressure around the rib cage.
- At the end of each full-body immersion, splash some of the cold water on your face or do a full-body dunk by lowering your head under the water. This completes the full-body exposure. Use this moment as the final transition period between leaving the stress and starting the adaptation process of warming up.
- After the full-body immersion, warm up naturally. The body will heat itself, which creates the adaptation phase. Don't disrupt the heat vent process by applying warm water or a heat source on the body. If you're very cold and uncomfortable, perform body-weight squats or jumping jacks to warm the body.
- After the full-body immersion, take slow, deep breaths to stimulate the vagus nerve and put the body in a parasympathetic state after the cold exposure. Inhale through the nose for five seconds, hold for one second, and then exhale for five seconds. Continue for 10 minutes.
- Following full-body cold exposure, sit or lie down. While taking deep breaths, hum or hiss on the exhalations as you create vibration in the vocal cords. This is a soothing breathing practice that stimulates the vagus nerve, promotes relaxation, and helps you bounce back after the stress of being in the cold.

Cold Urticaria

Cold urticaria is a skin reaction to cold. The reaction typically takes place within minutes following cold exposure. Some people have minor reactions such as swelling of the hands or lips, or temporary itchy welts (hives) on areas exposed to cold. Other people have severe reactions such as fainting, racing heart, swelling of limbs or torso, or shock. Consult with your doctor if you feel you are reacting poorly to cold exposure. Seek emergency care if after sudden exposure to cold you experience a whole-body response (anaphylaxis) or difficulty breathing (mayoclinic.org).

Extreme Cold Immersion: Open Water Cold Exposure

This last form of cold immersion uses bodies of water in nature, such as a creek, lake, or ocean, for cold immersion and is only suitable for athletes well experienced in the cold (see figure). First, you must understand the differences between cold water in a controlled environment and in nature. For example, in a shower you can control the temperature, and in a tub you can control the amount of ice used. In nature, the water moves, and this extra stimulus makes the water feel colder. The movement of the water creates a consistent "cold shock." If a cold tub is 40 degrees Fahrenheit (4.4 ºC) and so is the lake, the lake will feel colder because of this movement. The unpredictable nature of the movement can also cause your breathing rate to increase. For example, once you are sitting fully immersed in a creek, lake, or ocean and have calmed your system and slowed your breathing, a current can change and trigger parts of the body to feel a cold shock again. This will speed the respirations. Natural sources of cold water can also splash your face. These factors can add stress, and if you are not comfortable with or adapted to cold exposure, you might not enjoy this process, or it could be overwhelming and become unsafe.

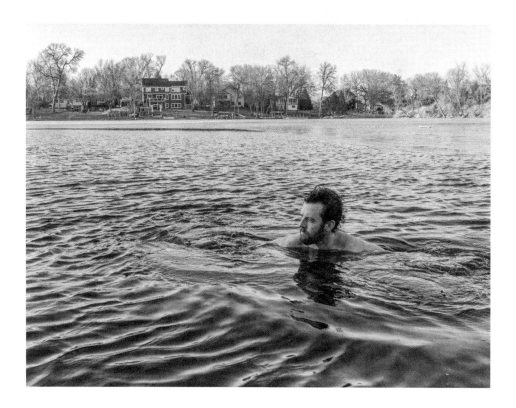

Cold immersion in nature is the best form of cold exposure because you reap many more health benefits and specifically benefits for the parasympathetic nervous system than in a controlled environment. This leads to not only physical adaptation but to mental adaptation as well. Being in nature decreases sympathetic responses. If you experience chronic anxiety or depression, spending time in nature will help heal the nervous system. Through the healing process of nature, you can rediscover your mental and emotional strength.

Cold-water immersion in nature should be done at a safe depth and in a weak current. When the current in a body of water moves you, the difficulty increases, and the current should not be strong enough to move you to a place that is unsafe. Make sure the water is shallow enough that you can walk out of it.

Cold-water exposure in nature is only available in colder climates and during specific times of the year. October to April in colder climates in the northern hemisphere are the best months to practice cold immersion in nature. The colder months of the year will result in colder water (December, January, February). It can be difficult to gauge the temperature of natural water, especially if the water has frozen over and you need to cut through the ice, so make sure the environment is safe and you are able to handle the temperature (see figure). For this reason, the protocols for natural cold sources are up to you. Two principles remain the same: (1) Warm up afterward naturally, and (2) the experience should be difficult, but never unsafe.

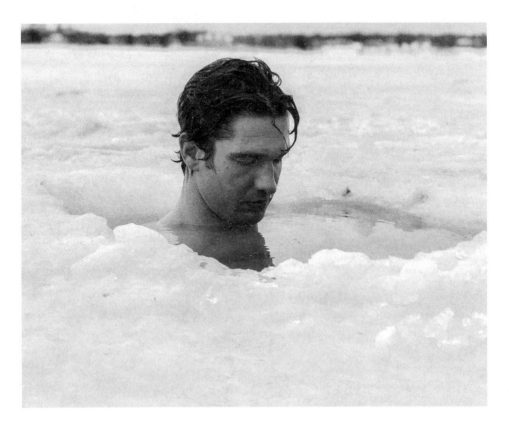

Mammalian Dive Reflex

The mammalian dive reflex is a physiological response we experience while holding our breath and being submerged underwater. Mammals maintain physiological homeostasis because of the nervous system's response that regulates heart rate, breathing, and blood pressure. When a mammal is submerged underwater, these checks and balances are modified. While holding the breath underwater, heart rate slows, and the peripheral vascular system constricts. The triggering of peripheral receptors allows the mammal to maintain oxygen levels. Major contributors that affect the system through the mammalian dive reflex are the nervous system, pulmonary system, and cardiovascular system. The primary result of face submersion is a reflex in bradycardia response. Bradycardia is a slower heart rate. By eliciting an increase in vagus nerve response, the body is temporarily placed into a parasympathetic state, and the heart rate slows (Godek and Freeman 2021). The benefit to athletic performance is using the built-in system to calm yourself. For example, between innings, periods, or halves, submerge your face under cold water to trigger a parasympathetic state and allow your mind and body to reset. Or before or after a game, dunk your head into cold water and hold your breath for 10 to 20 seconds to calm yourself and lower levels of anxiety.

General guidelines and time frames for open water cold exposure are as follows:
- *Beginner*: 30 seconds to 2 minutes
- *Intermediate*: 2 to 5 minutes
- *Advanced*: 3 to 7 minutes

Heat Exposure

This section focuses on the benefits that heat stressors provide to breathing, strength, and recovery. Although controlled heat exposure produces benefits for athletic performance, many athletes do not have access to a heat resource.

What Is Heat Exposure?

Heat exposure is what it sounds like: You deliberately expose yourself to heat. This section focuses on sauna heat. Other sources are a hot tub, steam room, and heating packs, but this book focuses on saunas. Heat exposure may pose more danger than cold exposure, so the rule of thumb used in cold exposure—"Whoa, I'd like to get out of this experience, but I can stay in safely"—has been adjusted. During heat exposure, you should feel relaxed, but once breathing becomes difficult and you begin to feel overly stressed or anxious, you should get out. If you have a sense you might pass out or feel claustrophobic, you have gone too far, and the heat is no longer safe.

How Does Heat Exposure Work?

There are limited ways to experience heat exposure in a controlled environment, so this book focuses on saunas (see figure). Saunas have been used for thousands of years and are still relevant today. Many cultures have used a heat source to help people relax, stay healthy, and unwind. Time in a sauna can mimic exercise: The heart rate increases, the body sweats, and the nervous system is slightly taxed. Sauna exposure increases blood flow to injured muscles and strengthens heart tissue. This section explores three types of sauna heat.

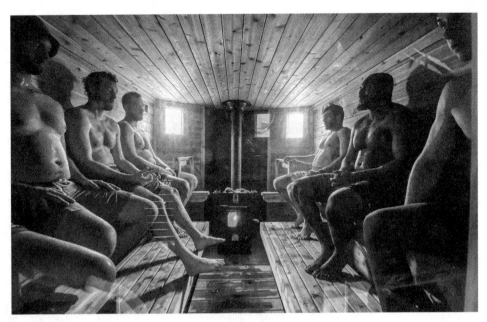

Wood-Burning Sauna

The wood-burning sauna is the oldest version and is still used. Many people become attracted to the wood-burning experience because of its authentic feel. The heat is generated naturally, and the fire creates a calming ambience within the sauna, lighting up the room and providing the relaxing sound of crackling wood and its smell as it burns. This type of sauna provides a soothing experience for the soul. Wood-burning heat is dense and deep. These saunas need enough ventilation to allow airflow into the sauna so the air is cleaner. The rocks on the sauna stove create steam when water is poured on them. This raises the heat of the sauna while intensifying the experience. A typical wood-burning sauna reaches 160 to 215 degrees Fahrenheit (71-102 °C). The temperature depends on how much wood is used.

Electric Sauna

An electric sauna is the most common and most convenient heat source. Most electric saunas are dry and unable to create steam; however, they are able to reach the same temperature as a wood-burning sauna: 160 to 215 degrees Fahrenheit (71-102 °C). If possible, find an electric sauna that can generate steam, which will mimic the traditional wood-burning saunas and intensify your experience.

Infrared Sauna

An infrared sauna is the most modern sauna and has become popular in athletics. The main difference between an infrared sauna and wood-burning and electric saunas is the maximum temperature. Infrared saunas reach temperatures of 120 to 140 degrees Fahrenheit (49-60 °C) and use a light source to generate the heat.

Smoke Sauna

No country loves the sauna more than Finland. This nation of 5.5 million people is home to an estimated three million saunas. And its longest-standing sauna practice is the smoke sauna (*savusauna* in Finnish). Whereas a typical wood-burning sauna uses a chimney to let out smoke, the smoke sauna has no chimney. Instead, a wood-burning stove fills the room with smoke, the fire is put out and the room is ventilated, and the remaining heat keeps sauna-goers warm during the session.

Sauna connoisseurs hold the smoke sauna in the highest regard. The heat is moist and the steam rises from the stove, filling the room with scents of smoke and birch leaves. During the session, bathers often use bundles of tree twigs called sauna whisks to slap other bathers lightly. This promotes better blood circulation, cleans the skin, and improves overall health.

Can't make it to Finland? Smoke saunas are popping up in other parts of the world.

Now that you know there are three main types of saunas, the question is "Which is the best?" The purpose of using a sauna to introduce heat stress is to challenge your breathing. The lower temperature of the infrared sauna doesn't cause enough stress to force breath control. Even though infrared saunas are a great tool for recovering and relaxing, they don't cause enough stress to reap physiological and psychological benefits. An electric or wood-burning sauna will drive both mental and physical adaptations through the release of norepinephrine and elevated heart rate. The adrenaline produced in response to greater heat forces you to focus on your breathing to remain calm. These are the same training effects produced by cold stimulus. And just as a cold shower is good, but a cold tub is better, an infrared sauna is good, but a wood-burning or electric sauna is better.

What Are the Benefits of Heat Exposure?

Heat exposure through the use of a sauna provides a variety of benefits to athletes that affect recovery, physical strength, and mental strength. They include the following.

- Improved overall health and life span
- Improved mental endurance, focus, and attention
- Reduced anxiety and chronic fatigue
- Reduced general inflammation
- Improved cardiovascular health
- Improved blood pressure

Rhonda Patrick, who holds a PhD in biomedical science, is a health researcher who has focused on frequent sauna bathing. (You can see many of her research articles at her website, FoundMyFitness.com.) Dr. Patrick's work has produced many findings and provided protocols for productive sauna exposure. For example, four to seven times per week, 174 degrees Fahrenheit (78.8 °C) for 20 minutes is associated with 50 percent lower risk for fatal heart disease, 60 percent lower risk for sudden cardiac death, and 51 percent lower risk for stroke. Furthermore, a single sauna session lowers blood pressure and improves heart rate variability. Other research has found that longevity is produced through two or three sauna exposures a week and is associated with 24 percent lower all-cause mortality. Using a sauna four to seven times per week is associated with 40 percent lower all-cause mortality (Laukkanen et al. 2015).

Controlled heat stress can also prevent muscle loss by triggering the release of heat shock proteins that eliminate free radicals, support antioxidant production, and repair damaged proteins in the muscle. Sauna exposure also increases blood flow to skeletal muscles, which fuels them with glucose, amino acids, and oxygen while removing metabolic by-products like lactic acid and calcium ions.

What Are the Safety Concerns of Heat Exposure?

When exposing yourself to heat stressors, you must respect the heat. Consult a physician before using the sauna for training or recovering, and make sure you understand the extent to which your body can handle heat stress. Just as your body must adapt to cold exposure and work its way up to handling longer times and colder temperatures, it goes through a similar process during heat exposure. Very few heart attacks or sudden deaths occur in saunas, but people who have coronary heart disease or have had a heart attack must be monitored and cleared before using a sauna. Using a sauna can be stressful on the heart and taxing on the body because it mimics moderate- to high-intensity training.

If at any time you feel sick, nauseated, or as though you might pass out, leave the sauna immediately. You may also be dehydrated, in which case the sauna impairs athletic performance.

Heat Exposure Exercises

The sauna should be used only as a performance-enhancing tool, meaning you should feel relaxed and rejuvenated after a sauna session. You will also notice better aerobic capacity, sustained energy, and a lower respiratory rate.

Before you begin sauna heat-exposure protocols, you should know a few things:

- Men should be shirtless and wear athletic shorts, and women should wear a sports bra and athletic shorts.
- Weigh yourself both before and after using a sauna. You should not lose more than three pounds (1.4 kilogram) in a sauna session. If you have lost more than this, you are headed into dehydration and should drink water immediately after the session and for the next several hours.
- Enter the sauna at a normal resting heart rate. (Chapter 5 explains how to determine your resting heart rate.) Monitor your heart rate while you're in the sauna. Heat exposure will mimic aerobic exercise and elevate the heart rate. If you are on a recovery day, maintain a low heart rate in the sauna. If you are on a training day, you can double your resting heart rate while sitting in the heat. For example, if your resting heart rate is 60 beats per minute, it may increase to 120 while sitting in a sauna at the end of your session.
- Once you're out of the sauna, sit for 5 to 10 minutes and breathe slowly through your nose to return your heart rate to normal.

Sauna: Heat Only

There is no specific preparation for entering a sauna. There is no need to perform breathing techniques before entering the sauna, as you do for the cold. Sit in a natural posture that supports healthy breathing and focus on getting used to the heat. Focus on slow nasal breathing and use the time as a form of meditation and relaxation. While in the sauna, you can perform any breathing practice from previous chapters that promotes relaxation, strengthens the diaphragm, or expands the rib cage. Keep these practices low stress. The breathing should remain slow and controlled, with short holds to slight pauses between inhalation and exhalation. Do not perform breath work in the sauna that is fast or uses extended breath holds that raise the heart rate. Besides that, it is as simple as sitting still in the sauna while you sweat.

Sessions are performed in rounds. On days you are training hard or competing, complete one or two rounds (typically one round), and on lighter training days or recovery days, complete two or three rounds (typically two long rounds). The guidelines and time frames are as follows:

- *Beginner*: 160-175 degrees Fahrenheit (71-79.4 °C), 12-18 minutes per round
- *Intermediate*: 175-195 degrees Fahrenheit (79.4-90.5 °C), 15-20 minutes per round
- *Advanced*: 175-195 degrees Fahrenheit (79.4-90.5 °C), 17-25 minutes per round

Sauna: Heat and Cold Contrast

"Fire and ice" is a good description of contrast training comprising heat exposure from a sauna followed by cold exposure. When your body is exposed to the heat of a sauna, it is in the fire; when exposed to the cold, it is in the ice. In the heat of a sauna, the blood circulation increases and blood rushes to the surface of your body, and the blood vessels and capillaries expand as they attempt to cool off. In the cold, the blood vessels constrict, and the blood rushes away from your skin and toward your internal organs. As you go through these changes, you will notice the temperature change supercharges your circulation through both the vasodilation of the heat and vasoconstriction of the cold. You should notice an adrenaline rush in the cold and a sense of calm in the heat. This helps accelerate recovery by moving metabolic by-products of cellular breakdown out of your muscles and into your body's lymph system for recovery. During contrast training, the heat is initially relaxing and causes you to sweat, and then the initial shock of cold raises your respiration rate as your body begins the process of fight-or-flight. When exposed to the heat, your respiration starts out slow (like the tortoise) and waits for the body to begin vasodilation. The differences between the body's response to the two types of stress lead to deeper understanding of them.

Before a Fire and Ice Session

Before a fire and ice session, sit or lie down and perform 10 minutes of cadenced nasal breathing: Inhale for five seconds and exhale for five seconds with a natural pause after each inhalation and exhalation. After 10 minutes of cadenced breathing, perform three rounds of Wim Hof breathing (page 162). After three breath holds, perform another three to five minutes of cadenced breathing before entering the sauna. This creates space in your mind so you can enter the training stimulus with a focused nervous system and a small dose of adrenaline.

Ideally, you will have access to environments at three different temperatures: hot, room temperature, and cold. The room temperature environment is where you will recover after using a sauna or cold tub. Most health clubs and gyms have a room temperature space between the sauna and cold source. If you're training outdoors, you need a house or tent at a safe temperature between the sauna and cold tub. A safe temperature is typically what room temperature would be indoors. The cold exposure used in fire and ice is full-body immersion, so you need a 100- to 150-gallon (378-568 liter) tub or a natural body of cold water. If you do not have access to full-body immersion, you can use a shower or buckets of cold water between sauna rounds; however, there is no protocol for this.

Fire and Ice Protocols

When using a fire and ice session, start in the sauna and finish in the cold. While in the sauna, breathe slowly and softly through the nose only. As you transition out of the sauna, take three minutes to let the heart rate naturally lower before entering the cold source. In the cold water, control your breathing by choosing the gear (explained on page 183) that fits your tolerance to cold. Stay in the water for the desired time and breathe at the following rate: four-second inhalation, two-second hold, and seven-second exhalation.

General Protocol

For the general protocol for fire and ice, use the sauna temperatures listed on page 192. If you are a beginner, perform just one full round and feel the sensations that come with fire and ice before moving to the intermediate level. Intermediate and advanced protocols use multiple rounds. You don't need to complete more than one round during every session, but you should follow the time guidelines for each round. Here are the guidelines:

- *Beginner*: one round, 12 to 18 minutes of heat and 30 to 60 seconds of cold
- *Intermediate*: one or two rounds, 15 to 20 minutes of heat and two to three minutes of cold
- *Advanced*: one to three rounds, 17 to 25 minutes of heat and three to five minutes of cold

The guidelines are presented as a range. If the exposure feels good, use the second number as your target. If it is stressful, decrease the number of rounds or use the first number as your target. If you feel overwhelmingly stressed or unsafe, immediately stop the session and enter the room temperature area.

No Protocol

Glenn Auerbach, founder of SaunaTimes.com, supports performing rounds of fire and ice without a specific protocol and instead focusing on remaining in control of the mind, emotions, and physical abilities by maintaining slow nasal breathing. If you have a low tolerance to either heat or cold, you can use high-gear breathing through the mouth. Set a goal to introduce stress frequently enough to adapt to the point that you can control your breathing through your nose only. This will indicate that your abilities have improved.

Søberg Principle Protocols

Dr. Susanna Søberg, author of *Winter Swimming*, developed the Søberg principle, in which you always finish contrast training in the cold and always warm up naturally. Dr Søberg led a study that found great benefit in going back and forth between cold and heat. According to the study, optimal exposure is 57 minutes a week of heat exposure and 11 minutes of cold exposure (Søberg et al. 2021). These results inspired the protocols provided in this section and are similar to those used in the study.

Protocol 1

This protocol consists of one round of 20 minutes of heat and four minutes of cold performed three times a week. It is paired with low to moderate exercise such as aerobic training or weight training to reach the full benefits. Three to four extended rounds of Wim Hof breathing on off days, followed by meditation and one round of fire and ice, can also be used to promote a low-stress stimulus, simulating light training or used as a recovery modality.

Protocol 2

This protocol consists of two rounds. The first round is 20 minutes of heat and three minutes of cold, and the second round is 15 minutes of heat and two minutes of cold. This protocol can be performed twice a week paired with light movement or light aerobic training to reach the full benefit. Pairing this sequence with yoga is preferable.

Protocol 3

This protocol consists of three rounds in which each round is 20 minutes of heat and four minutes of cold. This protocol can be performed once a week to gain the full benefit. Use three rounds of fire and ice on off days or for supplementation on days of light aerobic training.

After a Fire and Ice Session

After all fire and ice sessions, sit or lie down for 10 minutes of silent meditation. Use this time to shift into a parasympathetic state and slow the breathing rate. This promotes the adaptation process and helps you mentally shift out of the training session. Use the alternate-nostril breathing practice on page 156 to return to homeostasis. Start and finish with breathing in and out of the left nostril only. This helps engage the parasympathetic nervous system and lowers blood pressure. It will also help you enter a meditative and creative mental space after the fire and ice session. Because going back and forth between cold and heat taxes the nervous system, your breathing needs to recover after the experience.

When using fire and ice in the morning or afternoon, warm up naturally after the final round. If you are using it at night and within two hours of sleep, finish your final round on cold and use warm water, ideally a shower, to heat the body. This will keep the body from running hot for hours after the session and eliminate the energized feeling while you are trying to go to sleep.

Fire and ice is a very long-standing practice that has been used across many cultures. Use the protocols and guidance presented here to support your personal journey and allow the heat and cold to help you gain more awareness of your breathing and improve your overall athletic performance both mentally and physically.

Bibliography

Chapter 1

Allen, R. 2015. "The Health Benefits of Nose Breathing." *Nursing in General Practice*. July 6, 2015. http://hdl.handle.net/10147/559021.

Blume, C., C. Garbazza, and M. Spitschan. 2019. "Effects of Light on Human Circadian Rhythms, Sleep, And Mood." *Somnologie* (Berl) 23(3): 147-156. https://doi.org/10.1007/s11818-019-00215-x.

Born, J., K. Hansen, L. Marshall, M. Mölle, and H.L. Fehm, 1999. "Timing the End of Nocturnal Sleep." *Nature* 397: 29-30. https://doi.org/10.1038/16166.

Catlin, G. 1882, 2018 reprinted. *Shut Your Mouth and Save Your Life*. London, England: Forgotten Books.

Ehrlich, P.R., and D.T. Blumstein. 2018. "The Great Mismatch." *BioScience* 68(11): 844-86.

Elsevier. "Photosynthesis Originated a Billion Years Earlier Than We Thought, Study Shows." *ScienceDaily*, March 6, 2018. www.sciencedaily.com/releases/2018/03/180306093304.htm.

Harvold, E.P., B.S. Tomer, K. Vargervik, and G. Chierici. 1981. "Primate Experiments on Oral Respiration." *American Journal of Orthodontics and Dentofacial Orthopedics* 79(4): 359-72. https://doi.org/10.1016/0002-9416(81)90379-1.

Hsia, C.C.W., A. Schmitz, P. Lambertz, S.F. Perry, and J.N. Maina. 2013. "Evolution of Air Breathing: Oxygen Homeostasis and the Transitions From Water to Land and Sky." *Comprehensive Physiology* 3(2). https://doi.org/10.1002/cphy.c120003.

Jerath, R., C. Beveridge, and V.A. Barnes. 2018. "Self-Regulation of Breathing as an Adjunctive Treatment of Insomnia." *Frontiers in Psychiatry* 9: 780. https://doi.org/10.3389/fpsyt.2018.00780.

Kahn, S., and P. Ehrlich. 2018. *Jaws: The Hidden Epidemic*. Stanford, CA: Stanford University Press.

Kahn, S., P. Ehrlich, M. Feldman, R. Sapolsky, and S. Wong. 2020. "The Jaw Epidemic: Recognition, Origins, Cures, and Prevention." *BioScience* 70(9): 759-771. https://doi.org/10.1093/biosci/biaa073.

Karolinska Institute. 2017. "High Risk of Injury in Young Elite Athletes." *ScienceDaily* October 18. 2017. www.sciencedaily.com/releases/2017/10/171018090923.htm.

Kubota, T. 2018. "Stanford's Paul Erlich on the Problems of the Modern Jaw." *Stanford News*, April 10, 2018. https://news.stanford.edu/2018/04/10/paul-ehrlich-problems-modern-jaw.

Mayo Clinic. n.d. "Symptoms: Shortness of Breath." Accessed April 19, 2022. www.mayoclinic.org/symptoms/shortness-of-breath/basics/causes/sym-20050890.

Raupach, T., F. Bahr, P. Herrmann, L. Luethje, K. Heusser, G. Hasenfuss, L. Bernardi, and S. Andreas. 2008. "Slow Breathing Reduces Sympathoexcitation in COPD." *European Respiratory Journal* 32: 387-392. https://doi.org/10.1183/09031936.00109607.

Sapolsky, R. 2017. *Behave: The Biology of Humans at Our Best and Worst*. New York, NY: Penguin Publishing Group.

Shwartz, M. 2007. "Robert Sapolsky Discusses Physiological Effects of Stress." *Stanford News*, March 7, 2007. https://news.stanford.edu/news/2007/march7/sapolskysr-030707.html.

Wertheim, J.L. 2021. "Tom Brady Wins the 2021 Sports Illustrated Sportsperson of the Year." *Sports Illustrated*, December 15-16, 2021.

Chapter 2

Fallis, J. 2021. "How to Stimulate Your Vagus Nerve for Better Mental Health." *Optimal Living Dynamics*. December 24, 2021.

Kia'i, N. and Bajaj, T. 2022. "Histology, Respiratory Epithelium." StatPearls January 2022. www.ncbi.nlm.nih.gov/books/NBK541061.

Lundberg, J.O., T. Farkas-Szallasi, E. Weitzberg, J. Rinder, J. Lidholm, A. Anggård, T. Hökfelt, J.M. Lundberg, and K. Alving. 1995. "High Nitric Oxide Production in Human Paranasal Sinuses." *Nature Medicine* 1(4): 370-373. https://doi.org/10.1038/nm0495-370.

Maniscalco, M., E. Weitzberg, J. Sundberg, M. Sofia, and J.O. Lundberg. 2003. "Assessment of Nasal and Sinus Nitric Oxide Output Using Single-Breath Humming Exhalations." *European Respiratory Journal* 22(2): 323-329. https://doi.org/10.1183/09031936.03.0001 7903.

Srivashtqava, N. 2016. "Breathing Part 3 – The 4 Diaphragms" *Yoga Anatomy*, June 12, 2016. www.yoga-anatomy.com/breathing-part-3-the-4-diaphragms.

Zaidi, A.A., B.C. Mattern, P. Claes, B. McEcoy, C. Hughes, and M.D. Shriver. 2017. "Investigating the Case Of Human Nose Shape And Climate Adaptation." *PLOS Genetics*. March 16, 2017. https://doi.org/10.1371/journal.pgen.1006616.

Chapter 3

Bassett Jr, D.R. 2002. "Scientific Contributions of A.V. Hill: Exercise Physiology Pioneer." *Journal of Applied Physiology* Nov. 1, 2002. https://doi.org/10.1152/japplphysiol.01246.2001.

Benner, A., A.K. Patel, K. Singh, and A. Dua. 2022. "Physiology, Bohr Effect." StatPearls August 2022.

Bernardi, L., Gabutti, A., Porta, C., and Spicuzza, L. "Slow Breathing Reduces Chemoreflex Response to Hypoxia and Hypercapnia, and increases Baroreflex Sensitivity." *Journal of Hypertension* 19, no. 12 (2001): 2221-2229.

Bernardi, L., Schneider, A., Pomidori, L., Paoluccie, E., and Cogo, A. "Hypoxic Ventilatory Response in Successful Extreme Altitude Climbers." *European Respiratory Journal* 27, no. 1 (2006): 165-171.

Bernardi, L., Sleight, P., Bandinelli, G., Cencetti, S., Fattorini, L., Wdowczycszulc, J., and Lagi, A. "Effect of Rosary Prayer and Yoga Mantras on Autonomic Cardiovascular Rhythms: A Comparative Study." Health Module, *British Medicial Journal* 323, no. 7327 (2001): 1446.

Bradley, H. and Esformes, J. 2014. "Breathing Pattern Disorders and Functional Movement." *International Journal of Sports Physical Therapy* 9(1): 28-39.

Brinkman, J.E., F. Toro, and S. Sharma. 2022. "Physiology, Respiratory Drive." StatPearls June 2022. www.ncbi.nlm.nih.gov/books/NBK482414.

Brown, R.P., and Gerbarg, P.L. *The Healing Power of the Breath*. Shambhala, 2012.

CK-12 Foundation. 2021. "Anaerobic and Aerobic Respiration." Last modified March 5, 2021. https://bio.libretexts.org/Bookshelves/Introductory_and_General_Biology/Book%3A_Introductory_Biology_(CK-12)/02%3A_Cell_Biology/2.31%3A_Anaerobic_and_Aerobic_Respiration.

Cummins, E.P., M.J. Strowitzki, and C.T. Taylor. 2019. "Mechanisms and Consequences of Oxygen and Carbon Dioxide Sensing in Mammals" *Physiological Reviews* December 9, 2019. https://doi.org/10.1152/physrev.00003.2019.

Dallam, G.M., S.R. McClaran, D.G. Cox, and Carol P. Foust 2018. "Effect of Nasal Versus Oral Breathing on Vo2max and Physiological Economy in Recreational Runners Following an Extended Period Spent Using Nasally Restricted Breathing." *International Journal of Kinesiology & Sports Science* 6(2).

Doyle, J., and J.S. Cooper. 2022. "Physiology, Carbon Dioxide Transport." StatPearls July 2022. www.ncbi.nlm.nih.gov/books/NBK532988.

Fornasier-Santos C., G.P. Millet, and X. Woorons. 2018. "Repeated-Sprint Training in Hypoxia Induced by Voluntary Hypoventilation Improves Running Repeated-Sprint Ability in Rugby Players." *European Journal of Sport Science* May;18(4): 504-512. https://doi.org/10.1080/17461391.2018.1431312.

Hamilton, A. 2022. "Endurance Performance: Choosing High-Intensity Training Wisely." *Sports Performance Bulletin*. Accessed June 24, 2022. www.sportsperformancebulletin.com/endurance-training/endurance-performance-make-intensity-work-for-you.

Hurst, J.H. 2016. "William Kaelin, Peter Ratcliffe, and Gregg Semenza Receive the 2016 Albert Lasker Basic Medical Research Award." *Journal of Clinical Investigation* 126(10): 3628-3638. https://doi.org/10.1172/JCI90055.

Litchfield, P.M. 2006. "Good Breathing, Bad Breathing: Breathing Is Behavior, a Unique Behavior That Regulates Body Chemistry, pH." www.breatheon.com/media/docs/Peter-Litchfield-on-goodbad-breathing-CapnoTrainer8.pdf.

McKeown, P. *The Breathing Cure: Develop New Habits for a Healthier, Happier, and Longer Life.* 2021. Humanix Books: New York, NY.

McKeown, P. *The Oxygen Advantage: Simple, Scientifically Proven Breathing Techniques to Help You Become Healthier, Slimmer, Faster, and Fitter.* 2016. William Morrow Paperbacks: New York, NY.

Melkonian, E.A, and M.P. Schury. 2022. "Biochemistry, Anaerobic Glycolysis." StatPearls August 2022. www.ncbi.nlm.nih.gov/books/NBK546695.

Nobel Prize. 2019. "The Nobel Prize in Physiology or Medicine 2019." Nobel Prize press release, October 7, 2019. www.nobelprize.org/prizes/medicine/2019/press-release.

Panasevich, J. *Nasal Breathing: The Secret to Optimal Fitness.* U.S. News. September 7, 2020.

Patel, S., J.H. Miao, E. Yetiskul E, et al. 2022. "Physiology, Carbon Dioxide Retention." StatPearls January 2022. www.ncbi.nlm.nih.gov/books/NBK482456.

Rajneesh, R. 2020. "What Happens When You Hold Your Breath?" The Ohio State University Wexner Medical Center. September 15, 2020. https://wexnermedical.osu.edu/blog/what-happens-when-you-hold-your-breath.

Singh, U.P. 2017. "Evidence-Based Role of Hypercapnia and Exhalation Phase in Vagus Nerve Stimulation: Insights into Hypercapnic Yoga Breathing Exercises." *Journal of Yoga and Physical Therapy* 7: 3 https:/doi.org/0.4172/2157-7595.1000276.

Trincat L., X. Woorons, and G.P. Millet. 2017. "Repeated-Sprint Training in Hypoxia Induced by Voluntary Hypoventilation in Swimming." *International Journal of Sports Physiology and Performance* 12(3): 329-335. https://doi.org/10.1123/ijspp.2015-0674.

Woorons, X., P. Mucci, J. Aucouturier, A. Anthierens, and G.P. Millet. 2017. "Acute Effects of Repeated Cycling Sprints in Hypoxia Induced by Voluntary Hypoventilation." *European Journal of Applied Physiology* 117(12): 2433-2443. https://doi.org/10.1007/s00421-017-3729-3.

Chapter 4

Biskamp, J., M. Bartos, and J.F. Sauer. 2017. "Organization of Prefrontal Network Activity by Respiration-Related Oscillations." *Scientific Reports* March 28,7: 45508.

Brown, R., and P. Gerbarg. 2005. "Sudarshan Kriya Yogic Breathing in the Treatment of Stress, Anxiety, and Depression: Part I - Neurophysiological Model." *Journal of Alternative and Complementary Medicine* 11(1): 189-201.

Cacioppo, J., S. Cacioppo, and J. Gollan. 2014. "The Negativity Bias: Conceptualization, Quantification, and Individual Differences." *Behavioral and Brain Sciences* 37(3): 309-310. https://doi.org/10.1017/S0140525X13002537.

Chen, L., A. Becket, A. Verma, and D.A. Feinberg. 2015. "Dynamics of Respiratory and Cardiac CSF Motion Revealed With Real-Time Simultaneous Multi-Slice EPI Velocity Phase Contrast Imaging." *Neuroimage* 122: 281-287.

Delaidelli, A., and A. Moiraghi. 2017. "Respiration: A New Mechanism for CSF Circulation?" *Journal of Neuroscience* 37(30): 7076-7078.

Dreha-Kulaczewski, S., A. Joseph, K.-D. Merboldt, H.-C. Ludwig, J. Gärtner, and J. Frahm. 2015. "Inspiration Is the Major Regulator of Human CSF Flow." *Journal of Neuroscience Research* 35: 2485-2491.

Dreha-Kulaczewski, S., A. Joseph, K.-D. Merboldt, H.-C. Ludwig, J. Gärtner, and J. Frahm. 2017. "Identification of the Upward Movement of Human CSF in Vivo and Its Relation to the Brain Venous System." *Journal of Neuroscience Research* 37: 2395-2402.

Heck, D.H., S.S. McAfee, Y. Liu, A. Babajani-Feremi, R. Rezaie, W.J. Freeman, J.W. Wheless et al. 2016. "Breathing as a Fundamental Rhythm of Brain Function." *Frontiers in Neural Circuits* 10: 115.

Herrero, J.L., S. Khuvis, E. Yeagle, M. Cerf, and A.D. Mehta. 2018. "Breathing Above the Brain Stem: Volitional Control and Attentional Modulation in Humans." *Journal of Neurophysiology* 119(1): 145-159.

Homma, I., and Y. Masaoka. 2008. "Breathing Rhythms and Emotions." *Experimental Physiology* 93(9): 1011-1021.

Jung, J.-Y., and C.-K. Kang. 2021. "Investigation on the Effect of Oral Breathing on Cognitive Activity Using Functional Brain Imaging." *Healthcare* 9(6): 645. https://doi.org/10.3390/healthcare9060645.

Karavidas, M.K., P.M. Lehrer, E. Vaschillo, B. Vaschillo, H. Marin, S. Buyske, I. Malinovsky, D. Radvanski, and A. Hassett. 2007. "Preliminary Results of an Open-Label Study of Heart Rate Variability Biofeedback for the Treatment of Major Depression." *Applied Psychophysiology and Biofeedback* 32: 19-30.

Lippi, G., M. Franchini, G.L. Salvagno, and G.C. Guidi. 2006. "Biochemistry, Physiology, and Complications of Blood Doping: Facts and Speculation." *Critical Reviews in Clinical Laboratory Sciences* 43(4): 349-91.

Panchal, N., R. Kamal, C. Cox., and R. Garfield. 2021. "The Implications of COVID-19 for Mental Health and Substance Use." Kaiser Family Foundation February 10, 2021. www.kff.org/coronavirus-covid-19/issue-brief/the-implications-of-covid-19-for-mental-health-and-substance-use.

Reynolds, B. "There's A Lot of Uncertainty Right Now – This Is What Science Says That Does to Our Minds, Bodies." University of California San Francisco. November 1, 2020.

Robert Sapolsky Rocks. n.d. "Limbic System." www.robertsapolskyrocks.com/limbic-system.html.

Varga, S. and D.H. Heck. 2017. "Rhythms of the Body, Rhythms of the Brain: Respiration, Neural Oscillations, and Embodied Cognition." *Consciousness and Cognition* 56: 77-90.

Walsh, C. "What the Nose Knows." *The Harvard Gazette*. February 27, 2020.

Zelano, C., H. Jiang, G. Zhou, N. Arora, S. Schuele, J. Rosenow, and J.A. Gottfried. 2016. "Nasal Respiration Entrains Human Limbic Oscillations and Modulates Cognitive Function." *Journal of Neuroscience* 36(49): 12448-12467.

Chapter 5

Bellemare, F., A. Jeanneret, and J. Couture. 2003. "Sex Differences in Thoracic Dimensions and Configuration." *American Journal of Respiratory and Critical Care Medicine* 168(3): 305-12. https://doi.org/10.1164/rccm.200208-876OC.

Delgado, B.J., and T. Bajaj. 2021. "Physiology, Lung Capacity." StatPearls. www.ncbi.nlm.nih.gov/books/NBK541029.

Hallett, S., F. Toro, and J.V. Ashurst. 2022. "Physiology, Tidal Volume." StatPearls. www.ncbi.nlm.nih.gov/books/NBK482502.

Hamilton, L. 2019. *Liferider: Heart, Body, Soul, and Life Beyond the Ocean.* Rodale Books: Emmaus, PA.

Kaufman, K. n.d. "Understanding Student Burnout." NCAA Sport Science Institute. www.ncaa.org/sports/2014/12/10/understanding-student-athlete-burnout.aspx.

Lazovic-Popovic, B., M. Zlatkovic-Svenda, T. Durmic, M. Djelic, S. Djordjevic Saranovic, and V. Zugic, 2016. "Superior Lung Capacity in Swimmers: Some Questions, More Answers!" *Revista Portuguesa de Pneumologia* (English Edition) 22(3): 151-156. https://doi.org/10.1016/j.rppnen.2015.11.003.

Nicolò, A., C. Massaroni, E. Schena, and M. Sacchetti. 2020. "The Importance of Respiratory Rate Monitoring: From Healthcare to Sport and Exercise." *Sensors* (Basel) 20(21): 6396. https://doi.org/10.3390/s20216396.

Ontario Science Center. n.d. "Science at Home: Measuring Vital Capacity." www.ontariosciencecentre.ca/media/1170/scienceathome_vital_capacity_grade10.pdf.

Ranu, H., M. Wilde, and B. Madden. 2011. "Pulmonary Function Tests." *Ulster Medical Journal* 80(2): 84-90. www.ncbi.nlm.nih.gov/pmc/articles/PMC3229853.

Schünemann, H.J., J. Dorn, B.J. Grant, W. Winkelstein Jr., and M. Trevisan. 2000. "Pulmonary Function Is a Long-Term Predictor of Mortality in the General Population: 29-Year Follow-Up of the Buffalo Health Study." *Chest* 118(3): 656-64. htpps://doi.org/10.1378/chest.118.3.656.

Sharma, G., and J. Goodwin. 2006. "Effect of Aging on Respiratory System Physiology and Immunology." *Clinical Interventions in Aging* 1(3): 253-60. https://doi.org/10.2147/ciia.2006.1.3.253.

Skow, R., T.A. Day, J.E. Fuller, C.D. Bruce, and C.D. Steinback. 2015. "The Ins and Outs of Breath Holding: Simple Demonstrations of Complex Respiratory Physiology." *Advances in Physiology Education* September 1, 2015. https://doi.org/10.1152/advan.00030.2015.

UKEssays. 2018. "Respiration Values of Athletes vs Non Athletes." November 2018. www.ukessays.com/essays/physical-education/respiration-values-of-athletes-vs-non-athletes-physical-education-essay.php?vref=1.

Vranich, B. 2020. *Breathing for Warriors: Master Your Breath to Unlock More Strength, Greater Endurance, Sharper Precision, Faster Recovery, and an Unshakable Inner Game.* St. Martin's Essentials.

Chapter 6

Alkan, N., and T. Akis. 2013. "Psychological Characteristics of Free Diving Athletes: A Comparative Study." *International Journal of Humanities and Social Science* 3(15): 150-157.

Andersson, J.P.A., M.H. Linér, and H. Jönsson. 2009. "Increased Serum Levels of the Brain Damage Marker S100B After Apnea in Trained Breath-Hold Divers: A Study Including Respiratory and Cardiovascular Observations." *Journal of Applied Physiology* 107(3): 809-815. https://doi.org/10.1152/japplphysiol.91434.2008.

Cowie, R.L., D.P. Conley, M.F. Underwood, and P.G. Reader. 2008. "A Randomised Controlled Trial of the Buteyko Technique as an Adjunct To Conventional Management of Asthma." *Respiratory Medicine* 102(5): 726-632. https://doi.org/10.1016/j.rmed.2007.12.012.

Lynch, K. 2013. "Stig Severinson Sets World Record Double With Pair of Daring Freedives Beneath the Ice." Guinness World Records October 16, 2013. www.guinnessworldrecords.com/news/2013/10/freediver-stig-severinsen-sets-new-world-record-with-swim-250-feet-below-the-ice-on-a-single-breath-52227.

Chapter 8

Earthing Institute. n.d. "What Is Earthing." https://earthinginstitute.net/what-is-earthing.

Jovanov, E. 2005. "On Spectral Analysis of Heart Rate Variability during Very Slow Yogic Breathing." IEEE Engineering in Medicine and Biology 27th Annual Conference pp. 2467-2470. https://doi.org/10.1109/IEMBS.2005.1616968.

MacCormick, H. 2020. "How Stress Affects Your Brain and How to Reverse It." *Scope 10K*, Published by Stanford Medicine October 7, 2020. https://scopeblog.stanford.edu/2020/10/07/how-stress-affects-your-brain-and-how-to-reverse-it.

Miller, T., and L. Nielsen. 2015. "Measure of Significance of Holotropic Breathwork in the Development of Self-Awareness." *The Journal of Alternative and Complementary Medicine* 21(12). https://doi.org/10.1089/acm.2014.0297.

Sharma, V.K., M. Trakroo, V. Subramaniam, M. Rajajeyakumar, A.B. Bhavanani, and A. Sahai. 2013. "Effect of Fast and Slow Pranayama on Perceived Stress and Cardiovascular Parameters in Young Health-Care Students." *International Journal of Yoga* 6(2): 104-110.

Chapter 9

Cheung, S.S. 2015. "Responses of the Hands and Feet to Cold Exposure." *Temperature* 2(1): 105-120. https://doi.org/10.1080/23328940.2015.1008890.

Easter, M. 2021. *The Comfort Crisis*. Rodale Books: Emmaus, PA.

Godek, D., and A.M. Freeman. 2021. "Physiology, Diving Reflex." StatPearls January 2022. www.ncbi.nlm.nih.gov/books/NBK538245.

Kox, M., L.T. van Eijk, J. Zwaag, J. van den Wildenberg, F.C. Sweep, J.G. van der Hoeven, and P. Pickkers. 2014. "Voluntary Activation of the Sympathetic Nervous System and Attenuation of the Innate Immune Response in Humans." *Proceedings of the National Academy of Sciences of the United States of America* 111(20): 7379-7384. https://doi.org/10.1073/pnas.1322174111.

Laukkanen T., H. Khan, F. Zaccardi, and J.A. Laukkanen. "Association Between Sauna Bathing and Fatal Cardiovascular and All-Cause Mortality Events." *JAMA Intern Med.* 2015;175(4):542–548. doi:10.1001/jamainternmed.2014.8187.

Laukkanen, J.A., T. Laukkanen, and S.K. Kunutsor. 2018. "Cardiovascular and Other Health Benefits of Sauna Bathing: A Review of the Evidence." *Mayo Clinic Proceedings* 93(8): 1111-1121. https://doi.org.10.1016/j.mayocp.2018.04.008.

Mayo Clinic. n.d. "Cold Urticaria: Symptoms and Causes." Accessed October 13, 2022. www.mayoclinic.org/diseases-conditions/cold-urticaria/symptoms-causes/syc-20371046

Smith, E.N., M.D. Young, and A.J. Crum. 2020. "Stress, Mindsets, and Success in Navy SEALs Special Warfare Training." *Frontiers in Psychology* January 15, 2020;10: 2962. https://doi.org.10.3389/fpsyg.2019.02962.

Søberg, S., J. Löfgren, F.E. Philipsen, M. Jensen, A.E. Hansen, E. Ahrens, K.B. Nystrup, et al. 2021. "Altered Brown Fat Thermoregulation and Enhanced Cold-Induced Thermogenesis in Young, Healthy, Winter-Swimming Men." *Cell Reports Medicine* October 11, 2021. https://doi.org/10.1016/j.xcrm.2021.100408.

Wim Hof Method. n.d. "The Science Behind the Wim Hof Method." Accessed October 13, 2022. www.wimhofmethod.com/science

About the Author

Harvey Martin founded The Mind-Strong Project, where he has trained some of the top athletes and business executives in the world toward peak performance since 2017. Working alongside the player development staff in the Milwaukee Brewers organization since 2015, he specialized in training amateur and professional athletes from the NCAA, Olympics, MLB, NHL, and NFL in strength and conditioning, recovery, and mental performance. He began providing consulting services to universities in 2013 and would eventually teach at every level of college athletics around the 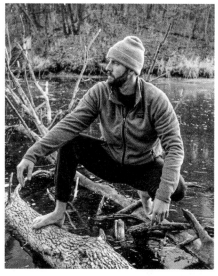 country. During this time, he helped develop culture and peak performance habits for over 1,000 student-athletes and coaches. Beyond the athletic field, Harvey has spoken and led workshops with Fortune 100 companies on how to optimize human performance and how to achieve peak performance habits with the use of breathing and mindset. In recent years, Harvey became the breathing specialist for the San Francisco Giants, where in 2021 the team set a franchise record, with 107 wins in a single season. Currently, Harvey is the human performance coach for the San Francisco Giants.

Harvey was a Division 1 athlete at Central Michigan University (2008-2011), where he received his bachelor's degree. He finished his playing career at Minnesota State University, Mankato (2012-2013), where he earned his master's degree while also teaching courses such as Coaching Theories, Strength and Conditioning, and Team Skills. As an athlete Harvey was a two-time All-American and was named National Pitcher of the Year before signing to play professional baseball with the Milwaukee Brewers in 2013.

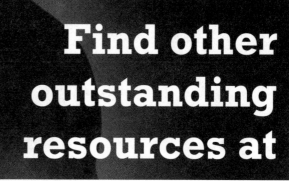

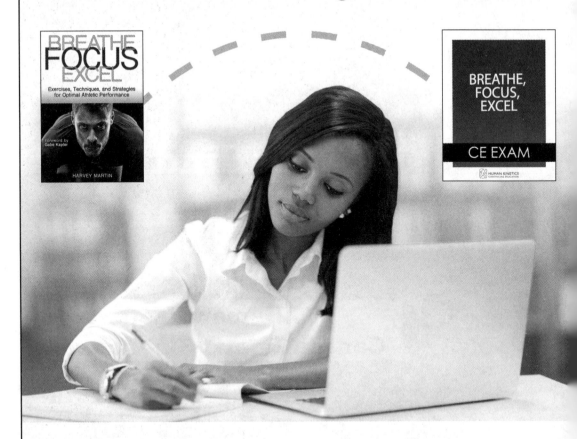
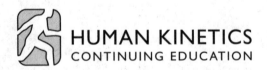